Energy
Healing
for Beginners

Also by Ruth White

Working with Your Chakras
A Message of Love
Working with Your Guides and Angels
Using Your Chakras—A New Approach to Healing Your Life
River of Life: A Guide to Your Spiritual Journey
Karma and Reincarnation

Energy Healing for Beginners

A Step-by-Step Guide to the Basics of Spiritual Healing

Ruth White

JEREMY P. TARCHER
a member of Penguin Group (USA) Inc.

Most Tarcher/Putnam books are available at special quantity discounts for bulk purchase for sales promotions, premiums, fund-raising, and educational needs. Special books or book excerpts also can be created to fit specific needs. For details, write Penguin Group (USA) Inc. Special Markets, 375 Hudson Street, New York, NY 10014.

Jeremy P. Tarcher/Putnam
a member of
Penguin Group (USA) Inc.
375 Hudson Street
New York, NY 10014
www.penguin.com

First published in 2002 by Judy Piatkus (Publishers) Ltd.
First Jeremy P. Tarcher/Putnam Edition 2003
Copyright © 2002 by Ruth White

Library of Congress Cataloging-in-Publication Data
White, Ruth, date.
Energy healing for beginners : a step-by-step guide to the basics
of spiritual healing / Ruth White.
p.   cm.
Includes index.
ISBN 1-58542-233-9 (alk. paper)
1. Vital force—Therapeutic use. 2. Healing. 3. Mental healing. I. Title.
RZ999.W483   2003   2002043573
615.8'52—dc21

Printed in the United States of America
3   5   7   9   10   8   6   4   2

To Sue Cross—a loyal friend, inspirer, and cotraveler,
with love, light, fun, and inspiration!

Acknowledgments

I should like to acknowledge and thank all who have helped,
inspired, and supported me in the writing of *Energy Healing
for Beginners:*

The individuals and groups who have come to me for
healing training, practice, and encouragement, and those
who have come to me for healing and counseling sessions.
The individuals and groups who have asked me all the questions that have manifested the information. My daughter,
Jane, for her unconditional love, support, and encouragement. The whole encouraging team at Piatkus, the original
publisher of this book. And my Jack Russell terrier, "Jack-
son," now eight years old, for his sense of humor and balance, and for his company while I type manuscripts.

Contents

Foreword

Although the concept of life energy is prevalent in Western societies, other concepts of the energy responsible for life exist in virtually all ancient societies. *Prana* from India, *chi* from China, *qi* from Japan, and orgone energy, developed by Wilhelm Reich, are all concepts of a universal life-sustaining energy. Paintings of Christ and of saints have usually included an energetic field around the individual, especially around the head and shoulders. This energy field has been called the aura, and it appears that about twenty percent of individuals actually see the energy field around people, animals, and plants, but an even greater percentage of individuals can feel this energy kinesthetically.

The concept of the *chakra* has always made sense to me because we do have collections of nerve cells and nerve plexi that are associated with the areas of each of the chakras as depicted in this book and other metaphysical writings. The first chakra corresponds with the sciatic plexus, the second chakra with the pelvic plexus, the third chakra with the solar plexus (and here, even the names are the same both in conventional anatomy and medicine, as well as in metaphysical literature), the fourth chakra is associated with the cardiac plexus, the fifth chakra with the cervical plexus, and the sixth chakra is associated with the brain. It is only the seventh chakra, our connectedness with the divine, that does not have an obvious physical component. In addition to these similarities in concepts of life energy and energy centers within the body, the concept of healing, or the laying on of hands, is also virtually a universal principle going back at least to ancient Egypt.

Some thirty years ago, I had the good fortune of meeting Olga Worrall, perhaps the most researched healer in history, and I became interested in documenting unique and "miraculous" healings. Over time, I received 15,000 letters from patients who wrote of their healing experiences. In over a hundred of those cases, where I had received permission from patients to obtain their medical records, physicians generally were unwilling to release the records to me. As one of my professors once said, "I am amazed at people who have eyes and see not and who have ears and hear not." The medical profession has been particularly resistant to the concept of healing.

Later, I had the great fortune to meet Ostad Hadi Parvarandeh, who provided me with over one hundred medically documented miraculous healings. Since that time, I have been able to demonstrate in one hundred and fifteen different individuals that healers working from a distance of up to a thousand miles can strikingly affect the electroencephalogram. This aspect of energetically affecting a delicate, scientifically verifiable aspect of human function is indeed one of the most striking examples of the potential effects of energy healing.

Dr. Elmer Green has demonstrated that an individual sitting ten feet away from a copper wall is radiating his or her electrocardiogram so that it's picked up by the copper wall. As we begin to see these unequivocal, scientific documentations of the effects of healers and even of our own energy on the environment, it becomes particularly important to pay attention and to treat our concepts of healing with the greatest reverence.

Ruth White has done so in this marvelous book, which not only discusses the broad field of human energy as it relates to the energy system and energy healing, but provides essential exercises for developing your own healing potential. I particularly enjoy her concept that it's possible "to develop and strengthen your energetic temple of being." She provides many tools for personal growth and healing of yourself, and for the concept of extending healing energy to others. She also wisely provides an extremely useful and accurate list of symptoms that require referral to a physician.

In many respects, *Energy Healing for Beginners* is not only essential for those who wish to begin their own healing journey, but is a great reference book with appropriate safe guidelines for all individuals interested in healing.

—C. NORMAN SHEALY, M.D., PH.D.
President, Holos Institutes of Health
President, Holos University Graduate Seminary
Founding President, American Holistic Medical Association

Introduction

"Hello, how are you?" is probably our most common greeting to each other—and exists in most languages. "I am well, thank you" is an equally common reply but often not an entirely honest one, since the greeting question is not usually an invitation to expand fully on our current state of health.

Yet the fact that the question is an integral part of every-day interaction indicates that how we feel in ourselves is important. Most of us know a condition of body, mind, and spirit that we'd describe as wellness. Equally, we're aware of various states of "not-so-wellness," from slight unwellness to definite illness.

Our experience of these degrees of wellness or unwellness depends on a number of complex factors linked to body, mind, spirit, and emotions. Honest answers to the greeting "How are you?" might include: "A bit liverish," "Rather down in spirits," "Very tired," "Quite depressed," or "Struggling with my emotions." Bodily symptoms may accompany emotional or mental states as well as spiritual malaise. All four ingredients intermingle, and when we first feel out of sorts we may not know which of body, mind, emotions, or spirit is the main contributor.

Of course, if we're really ill then bodily symptoms will probably prevail and we may need to spend some time in bed or consult a medical practitioner. When we're less than well or actively ill, we lose the ability to recharge our own fitness or energy batteries. We may need rest or relaxation of some kind to bring things back to normal, or we may need specific treatment and help. Increasingly, it is accepted that treating only one part of the foursome of body, mind, spirit, and emotions is rarely enough. In the same way, treating symptoms, such as headache or stomach pain, on their own may not deal with the underlying cause of an illness. In such a scenario, one symptom may disappear only to give rise to another. We're complex beings, and illness or malaise arises from complex interactions within us.

Fortunately, most phases of "not wellness" pass. Our powerful self-healing mechanisms kick in, and we feel better. We can truthfully and cheerfully answer the question, "How are you?" with "I am very well indeed, thank you." Sometimes, however, that self-healing mechanism fails us, and treatment of our symptoms does not make us well again. When this happens, are there other energies that can give our self-healing mechanism a boost and help us to trace a true way back to health?

I believe there are. I also believe that these energies enable us to move through disease—not simply back to a place of health we've known before but onward to a new place of health and well-being that's both different from, and better than, anything we've ever known before. These energies are healing energies, and are more commonly and freely available than we may realize.

HEALING IN EARLY SOCIETIES

Healers of all kinds have always been important to the continuity of human life. Even very early tribes are known to have had specialist healers, or medicine men and women. Many cultures have a special reverence for people who research the workings of the human body and who practice healing in its various forms. Early civilizations knew about herbs and other natural substances that aid healing processes or bring relief from pain. Although much early healing was ritualistic and employed the use of magic, there is archaeological evidence that complex brain surgery was performed by some of our ancient ancestors. Well-preserved skulls with neatly drilled holes have been found in South America, suggesting that there was early knowledge (later lost) of techniques such as trepanning to relieve pressure in the brain.

Every tribe had its healer. The young were carefully assessed to see which skills came naturally to them, and the healer was as important as the hunter or warrior. Knowledge was passed on from one generation to another in a form of apprenticeship. In Western society today, we have lost touch with the idea of looking for natural healing abilities in children—but, as we shall see in the course of this book, my work with healers has often brought people to me who have manifested a healing gift, and perhaps fulfilled a role as family healer, from quite a young age.

THE VALUE OF COMPLEMENTARY THERAPIES

Our present society relies heavily on the medical profession, as well as on scientific research, to provide healing interventions that grow ever more technical and complex. Yet in recent years there's been an upsurge in alternative or complementary therapies. Some people shun the medical approach and rely entirely on the alternatives. Others, including many doctors, think that natural therapies can be seen as complementary to the scientifically developed ones. This is a more sensible and sensitive approach. When complementary therapies are used in the healing process, it is more likely that each of those four important aspects of the being that interact to make us feel well or unwell will receive the attention it may need.

Natural therapies are complementary to one another, as well as to the conventional medical approach. Homeopathy or herbalism works alongside osteopathy or chiropractic, aromatherapy complements applied kinesiology, and naturopathy can be supported by reflexology. Many different combinations or permutations work well together. Doctors, surgeons, and complementary therapists all seek to heal. Pooled resources can have greater strength and lead to treatment of the whole being rather than the relief of symptoms on their own.

WHAT IS ENERGY HEALING?

Healers from all fields are usually very knowledgeable about the art and science of healing and make extensive studies of their favored approaches. They advocate specific interventions for specific conditions. There are also healers who know intuitively that they can heal by "the laying on of hands" or through working with the more subtle energy fields surrounding the physical body. Finding a title for this kind of healing is not easy. Some call it divine healing and draw their inspiration from a specifically religious source. Others speak of spiritual healing, which may be connected to a particular spiritual path, while others prefer to speak of energy healing. All work from a belief that there's a healing power that can be passed through one individual to another.

This belief has some foundation in the things we tend to do for each other when one of us is sick and the other well. We tend the sick. We hug or stroke a sick child or "kiss better" an injured or aching part. We smooth pillows, put a gentle soothing hand on a painful area, and prepare special foods with loving care. Such attentions are important to the healing process of the whole being. To be sick and alone is an unenviable fate.

There's a vast field between the natural skills of tending the sick (at which some people are recognizably better than others) and the wonders of modern medical science. We may not want to set up as professional healers, but many of us are interested in what we can do to help our own healing processes or those of friends and loved ones.

WHAT THIS BOOK OFFERS

This book suggests ways of extending and enhancing the natural skills by making us more conscious of them, as well as bringing greater understanding of the many interactive factors that affect healing and disease. It's intended to appeal to a wide range of budding healers, as well as to those already in training or practice. There's something here for you if you've ever wondered whether you have healing potential but have not yet explored the field, if you're a beginner on the healing path looking for more structure, or even if you're well established in healing practice but want to revise and rethink certain aspects of the healing phenomenon.

Chapter 1

I Think I Can Heal

Stella's story—What is healing?—Healing as a natural gift—
Can anyone heal?—Can I train myself? How do I begin?—
Making a start—Exercises—Establishing a healing flow

STELLA'S STORY

This story is similar to many that I've heard. Stella was the oldest of four children and already had two young brothers and a sister by the time she was six years old. After the youngest baby was born, Stella's mother often felt tired, or had a backache or headache. When her mother had to sit or lie down for a while, Stella would put a hand on her head, or gently stroke her back. It seemed quite natural to her to do this and very soon her mother recognized that Stella had a healing touch. She told Stella that her hands had eased the pain and afterward she felt like a new woman: calmed, re-energized and ready to do the many jobs her family needed, as well as to play with her children and enjoy motherhood.

Soon it was well known in the wider family that Stella had a gift for easing aches and pains, and soothing a fevered brow. Sensibly, her mother protected Stella from being asked to help too often or being regarded as different, special, or strange. Over the years, as Stella became more deeply involved in her schooling, exams, and getting a place at university, her gift was called upon less and less. There were occasional suggestions that she might want to study nursing or medicine, but no one tried to press her into a mold. Her own preference was for anthropology. While going to university, getting involved in reading for her degree, and then traveling for research purposes, Stella herself almost forgot, or perhaps discounted, her healing gift.

It was only when Stella married and put her academic career on hold to be a full-time mother that she chanced to pick up a book on healing. It made her think again about her early healing experiences. She had been shown at a young age that she had an aptitude for healing. Now she wondered whether the time had come to understand more about it.

Like many people, Stella didn't want to become a professional healer, but she did want to explore her healing potential. She wanted to know more about the nature of healing and find out how she could use a natural gift more efficiently, knowledgeably, and responsibly to help her husband, her children, and others close to her, as well as herself.

Stella had a number of questions. The first of these was:

WHAT IS HEALING?

This is the first question that anyone wanting to know more about healing is likely to ask. At one level, it's the most direct, simple, and obvious question, but anyone attempting to answer it must start by exploring what's in the mind of the questioner, for healing is not only an energy but also a process or journey. The journey enables movement from dis-ease to health. Channeling or harnessing the energy of healing can make that journey possible.

If the questioner has already shown a natural healing ability, they may ask, "When I put my hands on someone, what happens that is in some way different from someone else doing the same?" They're asking about healing as an energy or power. Questions about healing as a journey may come later.

Our bodies are, essentially, self-healing organisms or mechanisms. We have an immune system that helps us stay healthy and resist infection. When we get minor illnesses, like colds, digestive upsets, or a passing headache, we get better by a natural process. This process may be helped if we can take some rest when we feel off color so that our bodies can concentrate on coming into balance again, but for minor ailments we usually don't need to take medication or see a doctor. "I'm a bit out of sorts today—but I'll be better tomorrow" is a statement that reflects our faith in the ability of our bodies to recover.

When we get more seriously ill, something seems to happen to our self-healing process. We don't bounce back and we reach a stage where we know that help is required to make us better. We usually go to a doctor for such help and are given advice, perhaps some medication, and permission to take it easy for a while.

We might also look for help from the field of complementary medicine, where there are many different approaches to be considered. They're often based on ancient wisdom, and complement or offer alternatives to medication and interventions based on chemical formulae or surgery. Some methods, such as acupuncture, use little or no medication, while others recommend fragrances, herbs, minerals, vitamins, or food supplements. Homeopathy uses both natural and apparently toxic or disease-related substances in such minimal dilution that the contents of a finished homeopathic preparation are difficult to ascertain by scientific analysis. In the end, all forms of healing intervention have one thing in common—to kickstart the self-healing process.

HEALING AS A NATURAL GIFT

The sort of healing that Stella did naturally as a child has the same aim as any other kind of healing intervention: to help a body that is ill, in pain, or out of sorts restore itself to normality. Hands-on healers may sense some energy or vitality flowing through them and being transmitted to, and accepted by, the one requiring healing. Whether or not this energy is actually felt and identified by either party, this is what appears to happen.

What's the origin of this energy? Does it come from the healer in person or from some other source? The belief that healing comes from some other source results in it often being associated with faith, church, the divine, or religion. It's frequently called faith healing, divine healing, or spiritual healing. Such associations enhance its benefits for some, but can form a barrier for others who do not consider themselves to be religious or spiritual.

We don't have to be religious or spiritual to recognize that there are energies and forces within the universe that affect us both positively and negatively. If we think of our bodies as organisms that are, on the whole, self-healing, then it's not too big a philosophical step to imagine that there are forces outside as well as inside ourselves that nurture health and healing.

There are natural, universal energies that are, indeed, divine and spiritual in the widest sense, but which do not have to be directly linked to a specifically religious faith or belief. What makes a tree grow, a plant flower, a baby gestate and come to birth? There is something more than the seed in the earth or the meeting of ovum and sperm that perpetuates the process. So also with healing and recovery from disease, there is something "other" involved in the process. If that "other" can be harnessed, then we can help our own and our fellow human beings' healing process.

There are healers, sometimes called magnetic healers, who consciously build up their own vitality and then allow the one being healed to draw on what has been built up. For them, the giving of healing can be a draining, devitalizing experience, and they need time to recharge before healing again or even before going about the business of normal, everyday life.

For other healers, healing does not come from their own vitality. It has to be channeled in some way. These healers are able to let that something "other" that exists within the universe flow through them and into another. They feel vitalized, not drained, when they've given healing.

A rather mundane analogy for the process of healing via a healer is that of a flat car battery. It can be recharged by attaching jumper cables from a car with a healthy battery and allowing energy to flow through the cables into the flat battery. A magnetic healer might imagine being the healthy battery, connected to the depleted one and giving it energy. The other vision is to see the healthy battery as the universal source, and the healer as the jumper cables, providing a connection and a channel from that source to the flat battery, enabling it to vitalize itself.

This then, is healing energy most simply defined: the sensing of an available force that can be channeled through our hands to another human being (or an animal) whose self-healing mechanism is temporarily disabled.

Healers can, and do, learn a variety of energetic techniques and interventions, but many eventually return to the most simple—being a channel for healing energy. But, although this is where many begin and the point to which many return, the exploration of healing at and from subtle levels is wide and rich.

CAN ANYONE HEAL?

Through helping and training healers, I have found that, almost without exception, anyone who really wants to heal can do so. If the impulse and the desire are sufficiently strong to make you look seriously at even the simplest ways of developing your healing skills, something in you is urging you to recognize, use, and develop a natural gift.

In one sense it's true that healers are born rather than made: although training can help in directing, applying, and perfecting a natural gift, it cannot implant a basic flair or aptitude that's not already in existence. It's the same in most areas of life. I've been taught to play the piano and can do so well enough to amuse myself, but I'll never be a pianist because the natural bent isn't there. Some people take up a brush and paint beautifully with little tuition. When they're taught, their techniques, perspective, and artistic approach may blossom more consciously, but the basic gift is inborn. As in every field of giftedness, there will always be those healers who have an extra flair, but training will enhance natural skills, broaden knowledge, and increase understanding of the healing process.

Some people become aware that they have a gift at an early age, but those who haven't had such premanifestation but who nevertheless get a definite urge to look at what being a healer means should regard this urge as a prompting to explore something that's waiting to be acknowledged and brought to fruition.

CAN I TRAIN MYSELF? HOW DO I BEGIN?

It's possible to self-train, but the second part of this question indicates the need for some guidelines, some scheme to which to refer and, perhaps, a mentor to help you along the way. This book encourages you to use and develop basic healing skills, but if you want to train more extensively as a healer, then you need to find a course, a mentor, or an apprenticeship.

Initially, you may want to explore healing in a natural, simple way, mainly with family and friends. You may want to find out more about what is happening, both to you and your patient, when you're healing, and to learn what to do with your hands and thoughts.

People describe varied experiences when the healing is flowing through them. Some experience a tingling or a flow in their hands. Others may be aware of an infusion of energy coming from above them and down their spine, of a feeling of quietness surrounding them. Sometimes people feel none of these things and may simply have very mundane thoughts or conversations with whoever they are healing.

MAKING A START

It's important to do some simple energetic exercises to strengthen your awareness of energy flows. You also need a basic understanding of the subtle energy system. Many healers (given permission) touch their patients. Others touch only very lightly or work entirely in the auric energy field. Whichever method or combination you eventually choose, it is essential to broaden your experience and understanding of subtle energetic connections.

Training and practice give the healer the tools to interpret energy sensations received in the hands or the personal auric field as a session is taking place. The following exercises build from exploration, through preparation and rounding off, to a simple, structured healing intervention. They accustom you to energy flowing through you—like a warm-up. (It's a good idea to read to the end of the chapter before starting the exercises.)

Exercise
Sensing the Energy Field or Aura

This exercise is intended as an introduction to the complex subject of the subtle energy system, which is discussed further in the next chapter. Generally, the auric or energy field occupies a space of 4 to 6 inches around and beyond the physical body. It also interpenetrates with the physical body.

When you work with a partner in the way described in the second exercise below, you may find that you can eventually pick up each other's energy field at a much greater distance. When we're relaxed or in our own surroundings we fill more energetic space.

Working Alone

Rub the palms of your hands together for a few moments and then hold them about 3 feet apart. Gradually bring the palms of your hands closer and closer together until you feel a tingling sensation or slight resistance. This tingling or resistance indicates one edge of your energy field meeting the other, or the energetic poles (+ and –) interacting.

Working with a Partner

When you feel ready and there is someone else to work with, each rub your own hands together (as above). Facing each other so that the right hand approaches the left and vice versa, bring your hands in from a distance to meet those of your partner. Again, as you encounter the edge of the other's energy field, you will be aware of a tingling or slight electrical resistance.

GROUNDING AND ENERGETIC SEPARATION

You need to become aware of two basic principles of healing: grounding and energetic separation. These are important for would-be healers and must be practiced faithfully. Although the energetic factors involved in healing are subtle, they're also strong and require respect. It's all too easy for a healer and therefore the patient or receiver of the healing to become ungrounded, light-headed, and in an altered state of consciousness. For the transition from the healing experience back to the everyday world to be smooth and natural, grounding and energetic separation are essential.

Grounding or running energy (see exercise, page 16) is a preparation for healing. It strengthens your connection to earth, establishes a smooth flow within a central energy column running from head to feet and interpenetrating with the physical body, increases your sense of gravity, and gives you balance. During the process of instigating this, the healer becomes centered, calm, and receptive, a confident vehicle, enabler, and transformer for the flow of universal healing energy. A healer prepared in this way will already have an energetic effect on the receiver, who will also become calm, centered, and receptive.

In technical terms, this condition of receptivity and calmness occurs when our brains produce more alpha rhythms (as distinct from beta, delta, or theta rhythms). Maxwell Cade, a researcher of altered states of consciousness, biofeedback, and human potential who, together with co-researcher Nina Coxhead, wrote the book *The Awakened Mind,* designed a "mind mirror." When a healer and patient were connected to this mirror, it was possible to demonstrate how the brain patterns changed as the healer attuned, and how the patterns from the patient were then affected by this change.

Energetic separation (see exercise, page 19) is a rounding

off after healing. It's essential to round off or make an energetic separation if you're not to be affected, even slightly, by the symptoms of your patients. Healers in the very early stages of practice, perhaps when there has not yet been any guidance, often report a headache, or aching shoulder or knee, after giving healing. The presenting symptoms of the patient are mildly replicated in the healer for some hours afterward. (Sometimes these replica symptoms are mirrored: the healer, having healed a right leg, aches in their own left leg, for example.) Healers have to learn not to be blotting paper, and a properly visualized energetic separation is the principal way to avoid this.

Exercise
Grounding and Running Energy

Parallel to our physical spine, there is a central column of subtle energy. To maintain balance, groundedness, and good energetic health, energy should run freely through this column in two directions. (There is further reference to this central energy column in the sections on energy centers, or chakras, in Chapters 2 and 5, and in the illustration on page 17.) Imagining, breathing, and visualizing this energy flow helps it to be vital. Before giving a healing of any kind, attention to this energy flow helps grounding.

This exercise is also useful as a general relaxation technique or preparation for meditation. It's essential as a preparation for working with your chakras, which many healers do to strengthen their energy bodies (see Chapters 2 and 5).

You usually do the exercise twice: once in private, as part of the preparation for giving a healing, and again, more briefly, as a renewal, when you're standing close to your patient attuning for the healing. Eventually, as you gain confidence in being with patients, you might want to teach them this exercise and do it with them.

Once with your patient, you'd normally stand for this exercise, but in private you can stand or sit. Have your spine straight and your body balanced. Don't cross your legs if you're sitting in a chair, or your ankles if you're sitting on the floor (the lotus or cross-legged posture excepted).

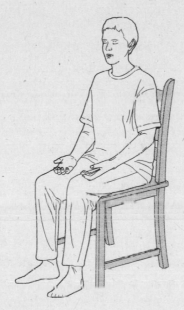

Relaxation position when patient is not present.

Nonvisual Method

- Begin by being aware of the rhythm of your breathing and letting it slow down a little.
- Now draw the breath in as though it comes from just above the crown of your head: draw it down through the center of your body, just in front of your spine; change to the out-breath at a point that feels natural for you, which will probably be around the solar plexus area but may be higher or lower; breathe out as though right

down and through your legs and into the earth. (If you are in a cross-legged or lotus position, the breath will not go down through your legs but straight out through your perineum area and into the earth, but these postures automatically balance energies in the body.) Breathe in this way about five times (i.e., five breath sequences; in/out = one sequence).

- Now, on the alternate breath sequence, begin to breathe, up from the earth, through the center of your body, letting the out-breath go up through the crown of your head. Continue to breathe in this way, without straining or forcing, for about five minutes. Always end on the downward breath sequence, repeating it in this direction more than once if you wish, as you finish.
- Feel the balance of your body and then proceed to prepare for and greet your patient, or to the giving of the healing.

Visual Method

If you like visualization and want to vary the exercise, particularly when using it as a general preparation for healing, here's a visual version. If the outdoor conditions are favorable and there's a suitable tree, it's good to do this exercise in a standing position, with your back against it and your bare feet on the earth. At other times follow the posture instructions given in the above exercise.

- Begin by being aware of your breathing rhythm. Let it be steady and perhaps slow it down a little.
- Visualize yourself as a tree. Your branches reach out above, your roots stretch deeply into the earth, your trunk is straight and strong. You're nurtured by the four elements: sun (fire) warms you and air refreshes you. Your roots are in the earth. They seek the underground streams and sources of living water.

- Breathe in through your branches, from the elements of air and sun, take the breath right down through your trunk and breathe out strongly into your roots, into the earth and the streams of living water.
- Breathe in now from the earth and the living water, bring the breath up through your roots, through your trunk, into your branches and breathe out into the elements of air and sun.
- Repeat these two breath sequences for five to ten minutes. Then gradually let the visualization fade. Feel your feet firmly on the ground, your own space all around you, and proceed with a sense of centeredness to your normal activities.

Exercise
Energetic Separation

This exercise is vital both to maintaining your own energetic health and vitality as a healer and to helping the patient use the received healing energy fully. During a healing, your energies mingle with those of your patient, and at the end, each of you needs to be firmly in your own energetic space once more. It should also be used after exploration exercises with a friend or partner (see pages 14 and 16).

When healing, you'll gradually learn to recognize when the healing flow is diminishing, but in any case, simple healing sessions shouldn't last more than twenty minutes. So either as you sense the diminishing flow, or as the specified time comes to an end, do the following:

Nonvisual Method

If you find visualization difficult, step back from your patient, give mental thanks for the privilege of the healing flow and, as above, drop your shoulders and let your arms hang loosely and relaxed by your sides, with your palms slightly curled and facing inwards. Say to yourself, "I enclose you in an egg of bright white light and myself in a separate egg of bright white light, with blessings on this energetic separation." The power of the words will achieve separation as effectively as when visualization is used.

Visual Method

- Step back from your patient, give mental thanks for the privilege of the healing flow, drop your shoulders and let your arms hang relaxed and loose by your sides, with the palms of your hands slightly curled and facing inward.

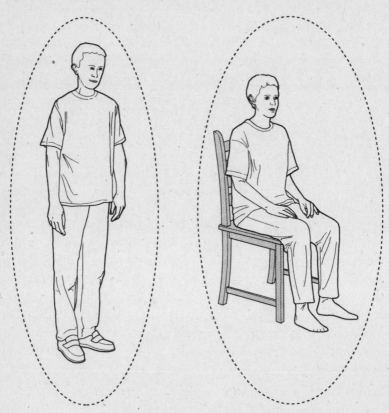

Visualization of healer and patient
surrounded by egg shape of light.

- Breathe in deeply from the point above your head and then out and deeply into the earth two or three times (always starting from the point above your head and not drawing up from the earth). As you do so, visualize your patient enclosed in an egg of bright white light (see illustration, opposite). Visualize a separate egg of white light surrounding you, and be aware of the space between your egg of light and your patient's egg of light.

Remember that these eggs of light around you ensure that you're each within your own energetic space once more. This procedure also helps both of you make a smooth transition back to the demands of normal life from any altered state of consciousness that may have taken place during the healing. The egg of light around the patient also ensures that the healing energy is contained, rather than dissipated, and will continue to be absorbed for as long as possible.

Exercise
Establishing a Healing Flow

For this sequence, I suggest that you find a cooperative friend with whom to experience and practice the previous three exercises. In essence, if the healer is well prepared and attuned, the healing starts, and effects are felt from the moment the attunement and grounding are complete. Although there are many other interventions to consider and learn, a successfully attuned healer is already generating a healing interaction. The exercises on pages 14 to 21 can be put together to form the basis of a simple healing sequence.

Begin by having your patient sitting comfortably on an upright chair, legs uncrossed, feet firmly on the ground. (If the chair is a little high for the patient, have a cushion or a small stool on which they can comfortably place their feet.

For reasons of grounding, it's important that the whole of the foot is flat and in contact with a cushion, a stool, or the floor.) Throughout this sequence, you don't touch the patient; this is a way of establishing the healing flow between two people.

Step 1

Standing behind your patient, begin by rubbing the palms of your hands together and sensing the meeting point between each side of your own energy field (see page 14).

Step 2

Remain standing behind your patient, and do the grounding and running energy exercise (see page 16).

Continue to stand behind your patient, sensing the calmness and flow that has come from the grounding and running energy, and encapsulating yourself and your patient in this flow.

Step 3

Make the energetic separation (see page 19).

This is the simplest sequence to establish a conscious healing energy flow between two people. The healer's preparation sets an energy flow in action and, when healer and patient are within that energy flow, the process of giving healing has already begun. The healer need do nothing more except the energetic separation for rounding off. The next chapters explore ways to build on this basic structure.

Chapter 2

Getting Started

*The subtle energy field or aura—Working in the energy system—
The chakras—Practical considerations—Carrying out a
healing session—Exercises*

The previous chapter described how to establish a healing
flow between two people. This chapter builds from this and
introduces touching the patient. It's important, even in informal healing, to have a sense of how you want to use the
healing energies to help your patient and to develop a healing sequence that has a rhythm and pattern to it.

A subtle or basic move forward from the sequence described
on page 21 is to step nearer to your patient at the beginning
of the session and hold your hands on or near the shoulders or head. This makes a stronger contact between healer
and patient and is already more personal and specific than
merely establishing a healing ambience.

Obviously, if your patient has an ache or discomfort somewhere in the body, it will usually help if the healer's hands
are placed on or above that painful part. Most patients want
healing for a specific complaint or symptom, and attending
to that is important within the healing sequence. Yet there

are other considerations that the healer using or channeling healing energy needs to be aware of, address, and incorporate into even the most simple of healing interventions.

THE SUBTLE ENERGY FIELD OR AURA

There's an energy field, or aura, around each one of us. The space we occupy does not end with the skin that surrounds our physical bodies. Our perception of what is going on around us is relayed to us by more than our senses of sight, hearing, smell, touch, and taste. If we're led into a silent, unknown room with our eyes closed, we'll sense whether the room is bare or furnished and usually get a good impression of its size. We sense when someone is standing behind us, not only because we hear or smell a presence but also because we're aware of a subtle response when others have stepped into our aura. This response may come as a slight shiver or tingle, or as a knowledge that a boundary around us has been crossed.

This aura is flexible. We don't have to physically take up all our energetic space—but most people feel happier and healthier in normal day-to-day interaction if there's space around them and if they know that other people are respecting that space. In a crowd, we need energetic space as well as physical breathing space. Most of us find crowds exhausting and demanding because when we're packed closely together our auras are forced to mingle. Under such circumstances, it's more difficult for us to "contain" ourselves than when we are alone.

In intimate and special relationships we share our energetic space with another—willingly, joyfully, or passionately—and benefit from that sharing and interaction. Crowds give us sensate overload that registers in our aura and we need time to recoup. Being in crowds or strange surroundings causes our auras automatically to draw more closely around

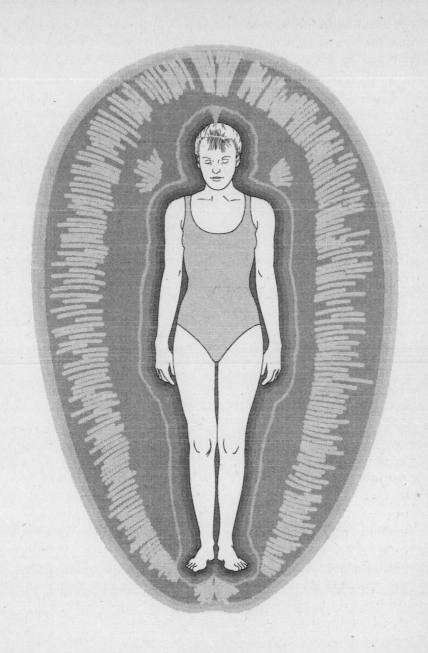

The aura.

us. People who are particularly sensitive in crowds and strange places may need to practice consciously gathering in their aura, so as to be more contained and less vulnerable to picking up too many impressions and energies from others at any one time.

The aura around us carries a slight electrical charge. Auras can be sensed and/or seen. People who see auras either sense a whitish light around others or see colors that change or vary with people's mood and state of health.

It may take a little training to learn to perceive auric colors, but many people can see the light of the auric field, given the right conditions. Ask a friend to stand against a well-lit, lightly colored wall. After a few moments of looking at and just beyond the line of body or clothes, your eyes may become slightly blurry with the effort of looking and you will see a subtle light around and defining the body shape. This is the aura. The development of an in-depth healing session is related to understanding the aura and its contribution to states of health and disease.

WORKING IN THE ENERGY SYSTEM

When healers work in the energy system, they work beyond the symptoms as well as with them and are able to discern the deeper causes of disease and pain. When the energy system is harmonious, the self-healing mechanisms within each one of us work more forcefully and enable our health-fulness. Allopathic (conventional) medicine and surgical intervention has often been criticized for being symptom oriented. It is natural to ask or expect any healer, allopathic, or complementary practitioner to take away the pain and discomfort. Yet there are often complex causes underlying the symptoms, the pain, and the disease itself.

On my wall, I have a chart listing the Bach Flower Remedies. It gives this advice: "Treat the person, not the disease, the cause, not the effect." Homeopathy is one of the complementary therapies that seeks to find constitutional remedies, and the same remedy is not necessarily given for similar symptoms. Chapter 1 presents a philosophy of disease and suggests ways of understanding the malaises that beset us more deeply. For now, it is enough to remember that, since we are basically self-healing mechanisms, the root of all our troubles, whether of body, soul, spirit, emotions, or mind, is that this self-healing faculty is underfunctioning. If it's given an energetic boost or triggered into activity, then natural healing could potentially set in once more and our recovery should be under way. In holistic healing, the self-healing mechanism includes, but is more than, the physical immune system.

Thus, at the most basic level, a healer working with subtle energies is aiming to reestablish the vitality of the inner tendency to self-heal so that the patient journeys naturally from disease—or dis-ease—to health. A manifestation of this may be that the pains or symptoms are eased. But healing should not be regarded as something that is necessarily immediate, magical, or miraculous. The movement from disease to health is a journey. The professional healer trains to accompany this journey with support, understanding, and, perhaps, more complex healing intervention. The non-professional healer, working with family and friends for the most part, seeks to invoke healing energies and forces so that the journey to health can be enabled. (All healers should aim to work cooperatively with whatever other treatment may be needed and should never seek to replace the advice and diagnosis of trusted medical practitioners.)

With this very basic intention of energizing the self-healing mechanism in mind, and with growing awareness of the nature of the subtle energy field, the healing session can be built into something that has shape, grace, beauty, and effectiveness.

THE CHAKRAS

Much of the color and energy of the auric field is supplied by subtle energy centers known as chakras. (The word *chakrum* is Sanskrit and means *wheel*. Properly speaking, chakrum is the singular form and chakra the plural, but in the West it's more usual to speak of one chakra and many chakras.) These are the points where universal energy enters and interpenetrates with our personal energy systems. For anyone able to see or sense chakras, they are wheels of light and color that both affect and are affected by the physical body. Most chakras carry links to specific parts of the glandular system and might therefore be described as subtle glands.

Nadis and Meridians

Another Sanskrit word, *nadis,* refers to the lines of force forming intangible layers and networks of energy that are the main substance of the subtle layers or bodies surrounding each one of us. The places where these lines or nadis are produced and at which they intersect are the chakras.

The major chakras occur where many of these lines are produced and cross each other. Minor chakras are formed where the crossing and production points are less busy. Nadis are tiny, sensitive energy lines. There are many of them in the energy field. Meridians are wider and more powerful energy pathways, but also originate from, and have crossing points within, the major chakras. A simple analogy is to consider the major chakras as major traffic circles in a roadway system, with the nadis as minor roads and the meridians as major roads.

The Locations of the Chakras

There are "echoes" of all the chakras in the palms of the hands. Flexing the hands awakens, or opens, these chakras, sets their energy buzzing, and enables you to experience your own subtle energy activity (see "Sensing the Energy Field or Aura," page 14). Healers use their hands to balance chakra and auric energies in order to activate the patient's self-healing mechanisms.

There's more reference to the subtle energy system (often referred to as subtle anatomy) in Chapter 6, but to get started the nonprofessional healer need only know where the chakras are located. The illustration on the next page shows eight chakra points and their positions in relation to the physical body. In descending order, the chakras are called: crown, brow, alter major, throat, heart, solar plexus, sacral, and root. The names don't need to be memorized. Working without too much theoretical knowledge gives you the opportunity to develop your own impressions and instincts in relation to each chakra and aspect of the energy field.

The chakras are major places where blocks form in our energy systems. If we learn to sense where they are and what they feel like, we can discern where or how they are out of balance and focus healing into these specific points.

Chakra Petals and Stems

In esoteric teachings, there's sometimes a lack of agreement as to whether chakras are situated in the front or the back of the body and its auric field. Some systems place them at the front and some at the back. The illustration on page 30 depicts the way in which chakras exist both in the energy field and in interpenetration with the physical body.

The exercise on page 16 gives instructions for grounding and running energy. Visualizing the up and down breath awakens and energizes a central subtle column of energy interpenetrating with the physical body and running from the crown of the head to the perineum (the area midway between the anus and the genitals).

Each chakra has something of the appearance of a flower, having petals and a stem. The stems of the crown and root chakras are open and contained within the central column. The other chakras have petals opening into the auric field at the front and stems projecting into the auric field at the back.

The stems normally stay closed but the petals are flexible, opening and closing, vibrating and turning, according to the different life situations encountered. A healthy chakra is a flexible chakra. Where there is dis-ease, the chakra structures may become inflexible or actually blocked. Directing healing energy into the chakra areas can therefore aid physical, mental, and emotional health.

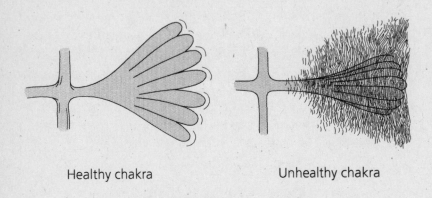

Healthy chakra   Unhealthy chakra

A healthy chakra has flexible petals that open and close.
A diseased chakra can become inflexible and
clogged, with darkened energy.

Polarities for Healing

The petals of each chakra are electrically positive (+) and the stems negative (–). Only the alter major chakra has a reversed polarity. In most people, whether left- or right-handed, the right hand will hold the positive electrical charge (+) and the left hand the negative (–). To balance the energy of the chakras, the healer usually places the right hand over the chakra petals and the left over the stems.

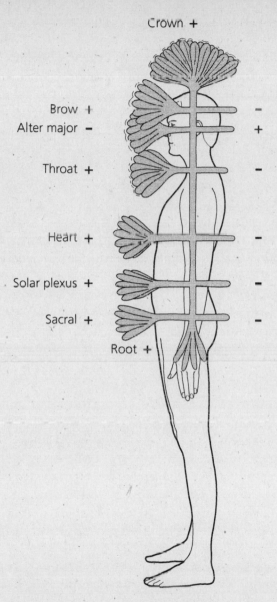

Crown +

Brow +

Alter major −

Throat +

Heart +

Solar plexus +

Sacral +

Root +

−

+

−

−

−

−

The seven best-known chakras, plus the alter major.
Energy flows both from positive (+) to negative (−)
polarities and up and down the central column.
Note the reversed polarity of the alter major chakra.

PRACTICAL CONSIDERATIONS

With some basic knowledge of the energy field, the nonprofessional healer is ready to make some practical preparations for a healing session. The professional healer often has a particular room or space in which healing is usually given. There will probably be a healing couch, and there will certainly be a chair on which a patient can sit, comfortably supported, to receive healing.

The nonprofessional healer usually has to improvise. It's unlikely that there'll be a table (of the kind often used for massage) available, and the best chair, in a home setting, will probably be a wooden dining chair or a kitchen stool. A dining chair gives back support and may be made more comfortable using cushions. A stool is, in some ways, easier for the healer, who then has free access to all the energy centers, but it may not be sufficiently comfortable or supportive for the patient. Whatever is chosen, it is important for the patient to feel comfortable in that position for twenty minutes to half an hour. For instructions on healing a patient who's lying down, see page 38.

To this end, as well as for reasons of grounding, a sitting patient's feet should be in close contact with the ground. Rather than have the patient's feet dangling or only the tips of the toes able to reach the ground, put a footstool or cushion under the feet and make sure that the whole foot is lying flat with both feet comfortably apart, and neither ankles nor knees crossed. (If the ankles and knees are crossed, the energy lines in the lower part of the body will also cross, thus affecting polarities.)

Since energy interpenetrates with matter, there is no need for the patient or healer to remove shoes, but it may be more comfortable for both to do so. In this event, attention should be given to keeping the feet warm—it's a good idea to have warm socks available. A patient may lose body heat during a healing session, and a blanket or wrap should also be kept at hand.

As a nonprofessional healer, you might need to treat a patient who's lying on a couch, or ill enough to be in bed. Once some basic techniques have been learned, they can be adapted to the circumstances. Beyond the simplest energetic healing exercises, there are others, only slightly more complex, that are particularly suited to patients who are lying down. One is given in this chapter, on page 38; see also "Drawing Out Negative Energy," page 134.

CARRYING OUT A HEALING SESSION

For your first attempts at giving a structured healing, it's best to have your patient sitting as comfortably as possible on an upright chair or stool (see page 32). If your patient has asked for healing of specific aches, pains, or particular areas of the body, check that they're happy for you to touch those areas of the body lightly when the time comes. Explain that you'll first be doing some healing in their energy system and that you'll attend to specific aches and pains toward the end of the healing session.

Genital areas are avoided when touching a patient, as are the breasts for a woman. Use your intuition about which areas to touch, in addition to any that have been specified as giving pain or trouble. You'll gradually develop an intuition or sensitivity about how long to keep your hands in any one place, but usually this will not be longer than five minutes. Applying pressure should be avoided and all movements should be very gentle. I've heard numerous complaints from people coming away from healings where they felt the healer was leaning on them rather heavily—so make sure you don't use your patient as a prop or support, and that you're well balanced or have a suitable stool on which to sit if the healing is a long one or you easily tire when standing.

Once you're carrying out full healing sessions, you'll need to leave time for talking to your patient both before and after a session. Beforehand, you'd discuss the reasons why healing is required, explaining what you're going to do, ask permission if you intend to touch the physical body as well as working in the energy field, explain that although the healing is usually conducted in silence your patient should tell you immediately if anything happens that is not comfortable for them, and that although the patient should generally be still, it's also all right to move or cry, or have an energy release.

Usually patients feel a great sense of calm when they're being healed and relax into a somewhat sleepy state. It's not unusual, though, for the healing to touch emotional levels held in the body—the patient may then shed tears, moan, move, cry out, make other sounds, or shudder. The healer may need to step back for a moment to allow this to happen or simply stay in gentle touch contact for a few moments longer than usual. Remember that the patient may need a tissue for the tears, and may occasionally interrupt the healing to have a glass of water and perhaps talk a little before continuing.

After the healing, your patient may need tea or water and time to return from the healing experience before going about normal life once more. This is the time when you can ask what your patient experienced and also report anything you felt or sensed during the healing session.

Your first practice healing sessions should preferably last no longer than twenty minutes, so bear this in mind as you time your movements from one chakra to the next. It means that no more than about two minutes should be spent in any one area of the body. You may sense an end to the flow into the chakra you're working on, which might come as a change in temperature or energy flow, an inner knowing, or an earthy awareness that enough time has passed.

Exercise
Healing Sequence 1, with Patient Sitting

If possible, practice the following healing sequence with a friend or partner before using it with someone less well known to you.

- Stand a little behind your patient, rub your hands together to activate your hand chakras and do the grounding exercise (see page 16). As well as being necessary to the healer's energetic alignment, this grounding is a preparation to allow healing energy to flow through the healer to the patient.

- Throughout the healing session keep checking that your feet are firmly on the ground, and keep your movements slow and deliberate, but light. Begin by working off the body, in the energy field: your hands will be about 4 to 6 inches away from the physical body.

- Hold both hands over the crown of your patient's head. You'll probably feel a tingling as you enter the energy field and you may be aware of a flow through your hands into the patient's crown chakra—but don't worry if you feel nothing at all. Many seasoned and successful healers simply trust and know that something is happening, without any specific subtle awareness of the process.

- Move so that you're standing on the right of your patient. (This is so that your right hand can easily treat the chakra petals, and your left, the chakra stems.) Hold your right hand over the petals of the brow chakra and your left hand over the stem. Keep a sense of timing and then move on to work with your right hand over the throat chakra petals and your left at its stem. (In your early healing sessions don't treat the alter major chakra. It has a different polarity and you can add it later. It's discussed more fully in Chapter 5.)

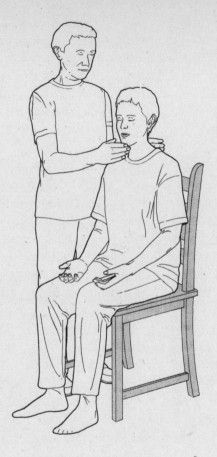

Healing the throat chakra.

- Move rhythmically through the chakras, right hand over the petals and left over the stem until you reach the root chakra. This should be healed with both hands, similarly to the crown, by placing your hands over the base of the spine or by kneeling down and placing them, palms upward, under the chair. (Throughout the healing session be aware that as energy passes though physical matter, you don't need to feel blocked by the back or seat of the chair.)

- Now—provided your patient has given permission—you're ready to begin touching the body. First, kneel at your patient's feet and hold each one in turn, with your left hand under the sole of the foot and your right hand on the upper part. Then, if your patient has any aches or pains or specific areas requiring healing, put your hands gently on or over each of these parts. As you get more confident in perceiving the energy flow, let the energy dictate the length of time you stay in each place. If you're uncertain, the general rule is not more than five minutes on any one spot.

- When you've finished this specific healing, it's a good idea to "comb" your patient's aura. You do this with the tips of your fingers, making long, sweeping strokes downward in the auric field, working from head to feet. This helps balance your patient's aura and also helps the regrounding process. Move all around your patient as you do this, beginning at your patient's right side and finishing off at the back.

- Rest your hands, from behind, lightly on your patient's shoulders and simply say "thank you." It's good to say this out loud, because it tells the patient that the healing is almost over. The final part is to stand away from your patient and make the all-important energetic separation (see page 19).

- Allow your patient time to begin to come back fully into the everyday world and, if possible, offer a cup of tea or glass of water. As you prepare these, you might like to take the opportunity to wash your hands as a final grounding.

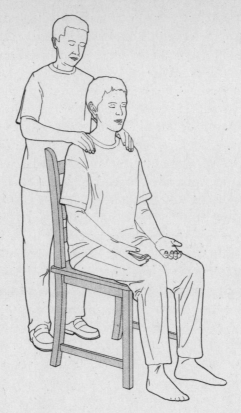

Energetic separation: Saying "Thank you" (see page 37).

Exercise
Healing Sequence 2, Patient Lying Down

This healing sequence is based on giving attention to the same energy centers as in the sequence described above, but it's used when your patient needs or prefers to lie down.

Often the only place to lie will be a sofa or bed, where there's very limited scope for the healer to move around the patient. If there's space underneath the bed and the patient lies near one edge it may be possible to heal the petals of the chakras with one hand and the stems with the other, but on many beds or sofas it's not possible to heal in this way without asking the patient to move around or change position rather often.

In general, it's best if the healing session is quiet, peaceful, and almost meditative. Asking the patient to lie first one way and then another, even if they're well enough to do so, is disruptive to both healer and patient. Try to have some reasonably free access to the patient's head. If they're not actually ill in bed, lying with the head at the foot of the bed or diagonally across a large bed can be a good way of accomplishing this. It might also be possible to organize a makeshift bed or mattress on the floor so that the healer, kneeling or sitting, can have full access from every angle.

The patient should lie on their back, with a pillow under the knees for comfort and support if necessary. Or you can heal the front first and, if it's comfortable for the patient, they can turn over halfway through the session. Alternatively, you might ask the patient to lie on one side. Eventually, if only one position is possible and access limited, heal where you can and trust that the healing energy will go to wherever it's needed most.

If kneeling is uncomfortable for you, as the healer, or you feel it to be ungainly in any way, it's best to either stand or sit on a low stool near the patient and to try to position yourself so that your back can be as straight as possible.

- Once your patient is comfortable and you have decided whether to kneel, stand, or sit for the actual healing, stand up to do your grounding and running energy preparation (see page 16). Then, if possible, sit, stand, or kneel behind your patient's head and gently focus on the crown chakra, using both hands in the energy field, as described in the first healing exercise (see page 14).
- As you work on the rest of the energy points, you can either use both hands over each, or you may prefer to

put your left hand on your left knee (with your foot flat
on the ground) and work only with your right hand. The
left hand on your left knee acts as grounding energy for
you, as the healer, and allows anything that the patient
may need to release to go into the earth.

- In this way, either using both hands together or keeping
your left hand on your left knee and holding your
right hand in the energy field over each chakra, work
progressively through the chakras—crown, brow, throat,
heart, solar plexus, sacral, and root. At the root, working
in the energy field, the position for your right hand is
roughly over the pubic bone. If you're able to use your
left hand at the same time, its best position for healing
the root chakra is over the coccyx.

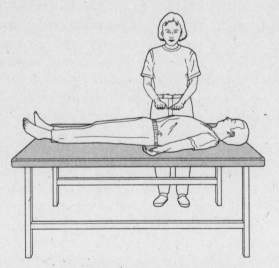

Healing a patient who's lying down.

- Now, if you can, place your right hand on or over the
patient's left foot and your left hand on or over the right
foot. After this, place your hands on or over any area
where there's pain or where specific healing may have
been asked for.

- Comb your patient's aura (see page 37), and then rest your hands either on your patient's shoulders or place them together under and cradling their head. As you bring the session to an end, say "Thank you," move away from the bed or couch, and make the energetic separation (see page 19). Allow yourself and your patient a few moments of silence before resuming normal conversation or having a cup of tea or some water together.

You've now built on the sequence that established a healing flow (see page 21) and begun to use the chakra energy centers for focusing the healing you invoke and channel. As you become more experienced, you may feel naturally drawn to holding your hands in other positions. Trust your intuition if this happens. These healing sequences are intended to get you started, not to be slavishly followed at all times. Throughout the book there are suggestions for different healing sequences and for elements that you can add to the basic pattern. It's important for you, as a healer, to have individuality and confidence in your work.

After a while you may become more sensitive to energies, but don't worry if you rarely feel anything. You can train your energetic awareness—and it grows naturally with experience. But always remember that some very experienced healers continue to feel little other than a sense of connection and a belief that they are instrumental in channeling healing energy. At some point, your patients are bound to ask what you've felt or sensed and may expect you to be able to say what your sensing means. If you're not a natural "senser" you can always turn the question around and ask what the patient's experience has been. The next chapter makes reference to sensations you or your patients may become aware of energetically during a healing session and discusses how to interpret this sort of information.

Chapter 3

Healing in Practice

Mark's story—How healers are perceived—Tempering patients'
expectations—Using invocations—The healing intent—Planning
and managing a healing session—Sensations to be expected
during healing—Using your intuition—Diagnosing illness—
Exercises—Structuring your healing session

Allowing yourself to become known as someone who can
give healing, even if only with family and close friends, can
cause reactions in yourself and others that need addressing
quite early on.

MARK'S STORY

Mark's experience was similar to Stella's (see page 7) but in
some ways entirely different. Mark's family also realized early
in his life that he had a talent for soothing pain and distress.
His gift was first noticed in connection with animals. He was
a tender-hearted child, particularly interested in nature.

The family cat, Bella, had always had a special affinity for
Mark. One evening she came home with deep gashes, prob-

ably from barbed wire, and had to have her wounds stitched. She was in pain, fighting infection, and began to refuse food. She lay curled up miserably in her bed, growing weak and thin, and not recovering well.

Mark was the only family member who could get a response from her or bring her any apparent comfort. He'd sit beside her quietly and then, without touching her sensitive body, gently make rhythmic stroking movements. This calmed the cat and she began to accept food again, first from Mark's hand and then, quite soon, finding the strength to get up and eat from her bowl. In a remarkably short time, from evidently having given up on life, the cat was well again, had her stitches out and never looked back, living on to a ripe old age.

Mark's parents felt great awe at his obvious healing effect on Bella. They were excited by what they saw as a special potential and giftedness in their son. They began to treat him differently, almost reverently, and told all their friends the story of Bella. It was not long before Mark was asked if he could help to heal a friend's dog. When this was a success too, he often found himself in demand when friends' and family's animals were injured or unwell. Of course, it was not long before he was asked to give some healing to an aunt with a migraine, an uncle with asthma, and a neighbor's child with an earache.

At first Mark enjoyed the attention and the novelty of sharing his new-found skill, but gradually he began to prefer to be out playing with his friends, racing his model cars, or watching television. He was a normal, fun-loving child, but his parents became quite obsessed with his gift and began to overprotect him and make him different from other children. He felt that his childhood was truncated from the moment he helped Bella the cat, and his relationship to his parents changed. He felt driven into an early rebellion against all things parental to claim an ordinary life for himself. He said, "I really believe something was getting quite out of hand and that if my parents had been religious they could have started some kind of cult, with me and my healing as the focus for it."

As it was, Mark's parents didn't really know what to do about his gift. They felt he had special powers but could hardly send a ten-year-old child to be trained as a healer. They did try to encourage him to study medicine or nursing, but Mark had been convinced from an early age that he really wanted to become an architect. When I got to know him, he had achieved that ambition. He was in the process of rebuilding the relationship with his parents that had broken down as a result of his rebellion and his leaving for a university as far away from home as possible at the earliest moment.

Although Mark had wanted to put distance between himself and healing and all that it had stirred up for him, he would never be totally mundane in his outlook. He'd cared for his spiritual side by becoming interested in transpersonal psychology (see Glossary, page 190) and doing a number of workshops. As he said, "I know that I do have healing gifts and I don't want to abandon them completely, though because of that early experience I feel quite dismayed by the archetype of healing."

HOW HEALERS ARE PERCEIVED

Archetypes affect us, personally and collectively, at almost every moment of our lives. By dictionary definition they are "primordial images inherited by all." Each human society is affected by forces such as peace, war, beauty, justice, wisdom, healing, death, birth, love, and power. The essence of these forces defies definition, and we need images, myths, symbols, and personifications to help us understand the depth and breadth of them. Tarot cards, which have ancient

origins, have twenty-two personified or symbolized archetypes in the major arcana. These cover most aspects of
human experience.

The archetype of healing, or the healer, is powerful
indeed, and all who practice healing of any kind need to be
aware of that power. When a profession, calling, or activity is
under the influence of a powerful archetype, it is necessary to
be in the right relationship to it. If we use archetypal energies
well, they can help us and even to some extent protect us. Yet
we need to be using the archetype—rather than be used by it.
If our own relationship to the archetype is comfortable, then
we can help others be comfortable with it too.

Mark had good reason to feel some dismay about the
archetype of healing. When his healing gift became manifest, the influence of the archetype affected and confused his
parents. Mark's childhood and his bond with his parents
became stressed as a result. He knew that he needed to know
more about the healer archetype before he could comfortably engage with his healing gift again.

TEMPERING PATIENTS' EXPECTATIONS

Hands-on or energetic healing is seen as a complementary
therapy that aids the whole healing process. Some people
fear healing or are superstitious about it, seeing it as being
related to magic. Others expect it to produce miracles.

Healers in professional practice usually have a high
proportion of patients who've tried everything in their
search for health or a cure and who come to healing as a last
resort, desperately hoping that it will achieve a cure where
all else has failed. The healing movement in our society is
growing, and there's no doubt that healing can and does
produce astonishing results some of the time—but not all of
the time. However, there will always be those particularly

outstanding healers who consistently produce extraordinary outcomes through their healing interventions and whose lives are completely rerouted as a result of the many and constant demands on them. Even when healing doesn't result in a cure, it almost invariably brings a sense of peace and relaxation, a changed perspective on disease, and a more positive relationship to the overall healing process.

What is expected from healing gets projected on to the healer. It only takes one or two publicized cases of uncommon results for a healer to become overwhelmed by public demand and for something akin to myth to grow up around them. This is the archetype of healing at work. Once a healer is recommended to others by someone who has benefited from healing treatment, the energy can build. People begin to feel better because they have a phone number and are going to make an appointment.

This is quite a weight for a healer to carry. Mark's (see page 42) parents were bewildered and overawed by the whole phenomenon and simply got it wrong. As a child, Mark was vulnerable and was swept along by something that no one around him could understand. Thus he became wary of the archetype of healing. As an adult healer, he knew that he needed to be in a position to fully explain his own vision of healing to potential clients and to help them understand what to expect from it—and from him.

The ability to do this applies to the nonprofessional healer, working mainly with family and friends, as much as to the professional. Too much build-up of expectation on the part of either the healer or the client will inevitably lead to disappointment or disillusionment. Seeing the movement from disease to health and well-being as a journey that the healer can support and accompany is one way of ensuring that the archetype is being used, rather than being allowed to take control.

Explaining that healing can help you to help yourself,

or your self-healing mechanism to restart itself, prevents patients from expecting instant results or from abdicating their own responsibilities on the healing quest. The majority of healings are not phenomena from another dimension, but the result of cooperative work between healer and client, usually as a complement to other therapies.

As a healer, you experience the urge to heal. Both you and your patients will want to fit this experience into some sort of belief system or structure. If you heal, you will ask and be asked questions about it, such as how you discovered you had the ability or inclination to heal, whether you do it as part of a religious faith or belief, whether you believe in miracles, whether healing drains you in any way, and what you feel, sense, see, and know when you are in the process of giving healing.

You may have a specific religious faith or belief. You may consider yourself to be on a spiritual path, or feel that because you can heal you need to find one. You may come from a humanist perspective. Whatever the framework, most healers regard themselves as channels or instruments for healing energy. Whether you take the most basic image for healing, in which the healer is like the jumper cables coming from a healthy car battery to one that is run down and needs charging, or prefer to describe the healing force as a universal energy or healing flow, without linking it to a religious or spiritual source, you'll need to align yourself with the healing energy.

The grounding and running energy exercise (see page 16) is also an alignment exercise, and adding an affirmation or invocation will help you to focus on your healing, your patient, your healing purpose and intent, as well as to become clearer about your healing role. All this will aid you when you're planning and managing your healing sessions.

USING INVOCATIONS

A good way to gain clarity of intention in healing is to make use of invocation, which is defined in *Chambers 20th Century Dictionary* as "the act or the form of invoking or addressing in prayer or supplication; an appellation under which one is invoked; any formal invoking of the blessing or help of a god, a saint, etc.; an opening prayer in a public religious service or in the Litany; a call for inspiration from a Muse or other deity as at the beginning of a poem; an incantation or calling up of a spirit; a call or summons."

Your invocation may be very brief or more complex and poetic. It's important that you feel comfortable with the wording and content of your invocation. As a non-professional healer you'll probably know reasonably well the people to whom you offer healing and may want to say your invocation out loud, thus involving your patient in this part of the preparation, or you may prefer to make your invocation silently.

The invocation can be placed at the very beginning of your healing preparation before you do the grounding exercise, or you may make it afterward as you step toward your patient and begin the actual healing sequence.

If you believe in angels or like the idea of angelic qualities as blessing and support for your healing, you can name them very simply as part of the words of your invocation. My book *Working with Guides and Angels* will give you more information about angels and about invocation. If you have a specific religion, you will probably use a form of prayer that you feel is appropriate to your healing invocation and intent. Here are a few simple suggestions for invocations that might be used by anyone as support to the healing preparation:

- I align myself with the power of healing.
- I invoke healing energy.

- I offer myself as an instrument for enabling healing.
- I invoke the angels of love, light, and healing.
- May I be used as a channel for grace.
- May we be receptive to the energy of healing.
- Thank you for the power/grace of healing.
- Let me be a clear channel for true healing.
- Let this healing be used according to the need of the patient.

Simple sentences are best, but if you want to put several together to make something more rounded or poetic, create your own favorite invocation(s) to become more explicit with yourself about how you view the healing energy and your role as a healer.

One suggestion for combining some of the sentences above would be:

> I invoke the angels of light and love and healing. I align myself with the power of healing in order to be used as a channel for grace. May I be receptive to the healing force and channel it with love.

When training healers, I always ask them to make a collection of invocations, some created by themselves and others gathered or extracted from other sources. Such an exercise helps greatly in defining and developing your ability to speak about healing and what it means to you.

THE HEALING INTENT

It may seem that healing intent can be defined quite simply as the intention to heal the patient of whatever is ailing them. Earlier I suggested that the main purpose of energetic healing is to kickstart the patient's own self-healing mechanism and to give support while or until this happens.

It is important for the healer to be clear about intent, both as part of relating to the archetype of healing, and also because thinking deeply about healing invocation and intent is part of the necessary process of forming a philosophy of healing. This is discussed in greater detail in Chapter 4, but I feel it's important to say that too much focus on specifics and symptoms in the healing intent can be limiting to both healer and patient.

Obviously, if a patient has a broken leg you'll both have the intent to use the healing to help the bone knit and to minimize any pain and discomfort. Yet even in such a straightforward situation as this, it's necessary to include in the intent a general healing for the patient and where they happen to be in life at the moment, as well as a specific healing for the broken leg and the pain.

Even a broken leg or other accidental injury can be a symptom. What caused the accident, both directly and indirectly? What emotional as well as physical upset and frustration is the patient suffering as a result of the accident and the incapacity? What contributed to making this accident happen at this time? Any injury or illness, however seemingly accidental or haphazard, is a part of the whole, wider picture, and the healing intent needs to be both clear and open.

If a healer is too attached to achieving specific results or to working with the symptomatic manifestation of illness or accident, something wider may be missed. As an everyday healer, you may protest that you only want to use a natural gift to be of help, so why make it more complex? Actually, this is right. Wanting to use a natural gift to be of help is an ideal intent, being simple, clear, and yet open.

If you want to expand your knowledge of how healing works and of the symbolism of healing and disease, it's wise to keep in mind the basic, simple premise with which you set out. Even if you go on to develop other skills to help where the journey to healing seems blocked, try to retain a simplicity of approach and intent, but one which widens, rather than narrows the framework within which you work. As you work with invocation and intent, let each of them reflect something of this simplicity and directness.

PLANNING AND MANAGING A HEALING SESSION

Gradually, a healing session will include much more than having a patient come for a healing, arranging them on a chair, bed, or couch, and conducting a healing session. Giving thought to invocation and intent will enable you to express your thoughts about healing more clearly and therefore to plan and manage a full healing session.

When planning a healing session, you need to remember that your patient may never have received healing before and may not know what to expect. It's up to you to put people at ease by explaining clearly and simply what healing is, and describing briefly what you intend to do during the healing session. It's a good idea to write yourself a script— not, of course, to read from when greeting your patient, but so you can see everything clearly thought out and know the words you intend or are likely to use.

Your patient, even if already well known to you, will almost certainly want to describe the history of their complaint and reasons for seeking healing. After listening to this, you'll probably want to ask what expectations your patient has of the treatment. At a first interaction, it's also a good idea to be clear about whether this is a onetime healing or whether you're going to meet regularly for awhile and then assess how things are going. If you have a long-term client, it's always a good idea to build in points of review, say after every four or six sessions, so that each of you can decide about commitment to further sessions. (Frequency of healing sessions is discussed in Chapter 7.)

If you have, or choose to develop, skills that are complementary to healing, such as counseling, you'll probably want to get more involved with the emotional and symbolic aspects of illness and spend time exploring these aspects with your patient.

Every healing session may have a different format from the last. You may intuitively use a different order of events or format for different patients, but on the whole your patient will want to know how long the session is likely to last, and there are certain standard procedures you'll need to incorporate. On page 54 there's a checklist for session management, including rounding off and completing the energetic separation by tidying and perhaps cleansing the space at the end of the session.

Preparing the Healing Space

It is ideal, of course, if you can set aside a separate room or contained space for your healings, but this will probably be difficult unless you eventually decide to heal as a professional. If you're fortunate enough to have a separate space, you'll need to keep it physically and psychically clean and clear, because healing has a subtle and sacred aspect to it.

Try to have color in the space, usually light, bright, pastel colors. Blues, pinks, greens, and yellows are all good (see the section on color in Chapter 5). If you're adapting a normal living space, a blanket, cloth for a table, cushions, flowers, plants, crystals, and candles in these colors will help you make the space more special.

Try to have two chairs of similar sitting height for you and your patient for the times when you'll be talking together. You'll also need cushions for feet, head, or to put under the knees of patients who may lie down on a couch or the floor. Rugs or light blankets should be on hand for covering and warmth, together with socks if the patient wants to remove their shoes. It's a good idea to have a jug of drinking water and two glasses, and a bowl of water and small towel with which you can wash your hands, both before you begin the healing intervention and at its end.

Cleansing the Healing Space

In preparation for healing your patient, the space can be psychically cleansed in several ways. You can use:

Sound. Music (Baroque is excellent); a shamanic rattle, singing bowl or rainstick (see Chapter 7).

Fragrance. A fragrant candle or an oil burner. Use this before your patient arrives, and put out the heat source for the oil before you begin the healing, as you do not want any fragrance to be too powerful during the actual healing session (see Chapter 7).

Smudge sticks. These are bundles of herbs that you light and then put out so that they smolder. You waft the resulting fragrance and smoke around the room and objects in the room to psychically cleanse and clear them. Smudging is a good way of attending to corners where negative energy residues may collect.

Prayer and invocation. As you prepare for your patient, you might say your favorite prayer or invocation in the room or space, silently or aloud.

Attention to and preparation of your healing space is also preparation for yourself. Allow time for it and do it carefully. When your patient has left the space, you may also want to repeat some of the psychic cleansing above, either in preparation for a new patient, or to establish a boundary between healing space and normal living space.

Session Management Checklist

This checklist will help you manage your healing sessions. When you're still at the practice stage, you may feel it's a little too formal—but it's best to be systematic right from the start. Even though you might leave out some elements in certain informal situations, try to incorporate a sense of ritual and thorough readiness at all times, out of respect both for the power of healing and for yourself and your patients.

Decide how long you'll need for a healing session. The shortest healing session usually lasts about twenty minutes. In addition, you'll need time for preparation, time for greeting and talking with your patient, and time for rounding off at the end. Never expect a patient to go too quickly from receiving healing to everyday activities, and encourage them to make sure that they don't have to get straight up from the healing space to drive a car, catch a bus, collect a child from school, etc.

1. Prepare your space. Make sure it's physically clean and tidy; gather your props (including blankets, pillows, and socks, as well as tea and water); and cleanse it psychically (see page 53).

2. Prepare yourself. Before the patient arrives, say your invocation (see page 48) and do your grounding and running energy exercise (see page 16).

3. Greet your patient. Know where you'll put coats, whether or not you'll ask that shoes be removed; offer refreshments (tea or water).

4. Talk with your patient. Ask what they may be expecting, and give an opportunity for any questions to be asked.

- Give information about how you'll conduct the healing session and ask your patient any appropriate questions about their reasons for coming
- Explain that you'll probably be silent during the healing session but encourage your patient to know that it is all right to speak, move, and react to the healing.
- Explain that extra pillows or coverings are available and that you'll want to know if your patient feels uncomfortable in any way, including about anything you do during the healing that the patient may want to question.
- Be clear about whether or not your patient is happy with being touched at the appropriate time in the healing intervention.

5. Prepare your patient for the healing session. Reground yourself, maybe teaching this exercise to your patient as well (see page 16); remind yourself of your healing intent and/or invocation (see page 48).

6. Carry out the healing exercise of your choice.

7. Do the energetic separation (see page 19).

8. After a little time, ask your patient to move from the healing chair or couch, offer more water or tea, and exchange what each of you has experienced during the session.

9. Make any arrangements that need to be made about future sessions. Make sure that your patient can contact you if they're worried about anything in the interim. Make sure that your patient has gathered all personal belongings. End the session.

10. Rearrange your room, play music, or cleanse the space as you did before interacting with your patient, leaving it ready for your next patient or for its normal use.

SENSATIONS TO BE EXPECTED DURING HEALING

As you practice the healing exercises suggested so far, you'll begin to feel or perceive things that are happening for you and your patient in terms of energy flow. You'll gradually respond to certain perceptions of what's going on. Where energy is experienced as "fizzy," you'll bring in the intention to quieten and calm. As well as an overall healing intention for your patient, you'll have intentions of the moment that develop in response to what you're sensing.

Knowing the meanings of the things you begin to feel or perceive as you're giving healing is something that can only come from experience, which takes time to build and is aided by working with different patients and their different symptoms.

Right from the start, it can help to have a "vocabulary list for healing" in mind, so that you know what you might be looking for and what the energy you're channeling might seek to rectify. Having such a list may seem like the beginning of crossing the boundary from complete simplicity to greater complexity, but as you seek to be more conscious as a healer, some movement from innocent trust to increased knowledge and deliberation has to be made. My hope for healers is that moving into greater awareness will eventually help them to return to a style that is relatively unadorned and might be described as "informed simplicity."

The Vocabulary of Healing

Here is the vocabulary list for healing (in alphabetical order):

agitated, alive, asleep, awake, balanced, blocked, blossoming, bold, bright, brittle, bubbly, budding, calm, changeable, closed, cool, cold, collected, complex, composed, consistent, dark, dead, difficult, distressed, dry, dull, easy, empty, excited, effervescent, electrical, faint, fast, fertile, fiery, floppy, flowing, free, full, gentle, gritty, grounded, growing, hard, harsh, healthy, heavy, hot, hungry, icy, immobile, inconsistent, insubstantial, irregular, jarring, joyful, jumpy, light, lively, magnetic, moist, moving, narrow, normal, nourished, open, peaceful, prickly, pulsating, quick, quickening, quiet, receptive, regular, released, replete, resistant, restful, restorative, rigid, sad, scattered, sensitive, simple, slow, smooth, soft, solid, spiky, stable, stagnant, static, steady, sticky, stiff, strong, stuck, substantial, sustained, tingling, thick, thirsty, unbalanced, undernourished, ungrounded, unreceptive, unstable, unsteady, unsustained, warm, weak, wide.

These words all describe ways of perceiving the energy in chakras, aura, and body. The list is not totally comprehensive, and you may want to add words of your own, but it is a starting point.

Words Describing Healthy Energies

Obviously, healthy energies will tend to be perceived as:

alive, awake, balanced, blossoming, bright, calm, collected, composed, consistent, easy, electrical, fertile, flowing, free, gentle, grounded, healthy, joyful, light, lively, magnetic, moving, normal, nourished, peaceful, quiet, receptive, regular, restful, restorative, stable, smooth, steady, sustained.

Words Describing Energies That Need Attention

Energies that are out of balance or needing attention of some kind may be perceived as:

agitated, bold, brittle, bubbly, budding, changeable, closed, cool, cold, complex, dead, difficult, distressed, dry, dull, empty, excited, effervescent, faint, fast, fiery, floppy, gritty, growing, hard, harsh, heavy, hot, hungry, icy, immobile, inconsistent, insubstantial, irregular, jarring, jumpy, moist, narrow, open, prickly, pulsating, quick, quickening, released, replete, resistant, rigid, sad, scattered, sensitive, simple, slow, soft, solid, spiky, stagnant, static, sticky, stiff, strong, stuck, substantial, tingling, thick, thirsty, unbalanced, undernourished, ungrounded, unreceptive, unstable, unsteady, unsustained, warm, weak, wide.

Sensing the Meanings of Different Energies

It will be largely self-evident that agitated energy needs calming, changeable energy needs steadying, cold areas need warming, dead ones enlivening, and hungry ones feeding, but there are also words in the list that may or may not indicate the need for change. If certain kinds of energy are perceived, the healer needs to sense further and maybe ask inner questions.

Overall, balance is what a healer aims to achieve or has as an intention. Thus, a bold energy can be positive, or it could be too bold and out of proportion to other energies that may be perceived. A bubbly energy might feel balanced and productive, recuperative and responsive, or it might be unbalanced. Where there is emptiness, there might be deadness, but there could also be a sense of clearance and anticipation. A perception of fullness might indicate near-blockage, or might be the fullness that precedes blossoming. Effervescent energy can indicate life returning to an area that needs to be encouraged, but can also mean over-activity that needs to be quieted. An open energy may mean that something has been satisfactorily released, but if chakras, in particular, are too open, depletion and exhaustion may be present in the patient. Similarly, a closed energy may mean that there is a healthy protection, but could signal resistance or a potential underlying blockage. Whatever you sense, you need also to consider its relationship to the environment, yourself, and your patient's condition. Your intuition is always your best guide and will naturally strengthen as you gain experience in healing.

Familiarizing yourself with these words, or choosing a few from the list to have in mind when healing, will give you a vocabulary for what you may perceive and help you to be more informed about what's happening when you heal. It may also enable you to be aware of areas that need more focus during the healing intervention. As your experience builds and your perceptions heighten, your sensing of what is going on will tell you more and more about the needs of your patient and enable your healing responses to be more specific.

USING YOUR INTUITION

As you begin to notice what needs to be achieved energetic-ally for your patient, you may intuitively begin to develop some particular hand gestures, or decide you want to use crystals, fragrances, or colors as aids to your healing sequence (see Chapter 7). When you're healing, your hands will usually be relaxed and slightly curved, with fingers together but not rigidly so. But now you may find that you're drawn to use only your fingers, only some of your fingers, or mainly the palms of your hands. Trust this.

Where you can, practice and experiment with like-minded friends who'll give you feedback, or look for a group of healers to join, where such things can be discussed. You may also decide that you don't want to do anything more than hold your hands over certain areas with the aim of achieving balance. Some people move their hands rhythmically, others keep them still—use your intuition.

The middle pathway between a relatively complex healing procedure and a very simple one is to note what seems to be happening in the patient's energy field and to know what you want to accomplish. Focusing this intention into specific areas will bring a natural direction to your healing and will be something to discuss with your patient after the healing has taken place and before further healing is given.

Involving your patient in the healing process is important. If you discuss what you've sensed and make suggestions for what needs to be achieved, your patient can keep this in mind between sessions and use it for meditative self-healing. (This is further discussed in Chapters 4 and 7.)

DIAGNOSING ILLNESSES

There are gifted, sensitive, mediumistic, or clairvoyant healers who can diagnose physical illnesses without recourse to medical science, but apart from knowing what's happening in the energy field and chakras, even professional healers are well advised to leave specific diagnosis aside. As your sensitivity develops, you may pick up on organs in the body that do not seem to be functioning well or that you suspect are diseased.

Such sensings need to be reported gently to your patient, without creating alarm and with the advice to visit a doctor to get things checked out. If you sense energy that's "stuck" in the liver, for example, it doesn't necessarily mean that the organ is diseased, but healing is best practiced as a complementary therapy, not an alternative one. When in doubt, both you and your patient may need expert advice. Also bear in mind that no one's energy field is perfectly balanced. There will be blocks, but most of these are fairly harmless. As you do more healing you'll begin to sense when someone is ill.

Rapport between doctors and healers can sometimes be fraught with difficulty. Doctors have legal obligations to their patients. Healers can be woefully lacking in tact and respect when it comes to imparting what they sense or intuit. It is well to remember that the majority of doctors enter the profession because they are dedicated to the healing of disease. They undergo many years of training and have sophisticated tools available for making diagnoses.

As healers, we may feel that medical science is too symptom oriented and not in touch with the healing of the whole person, or fails to give enough weight to what the individual may choose in the way of treatment. Thankfully, this is gradually changing and doctors' patients are given more information and choice. Many doctors' offices and clinics now invite healers to work with those patients who are open to it.

Cooperation between the medical profession and comple mentary therapies progresses where there is mutual respect. To aid this, it's best if most healers focus on energy imbalances and leave scientific diagnosis to those who are best trained and equipped to attempt it. Chapter 4 explains something of the deeper, symbolic level of symptoms. (Appendix, page 185, lists symptoms that should be reported to a doctor, if they haven't already been, before progressing further with the healing.)

STRUCTURING YOUR HEALING SESSION

Now you can begin to expand your basic healing technique with these simple steps:

Step 1. Invocations

Write some invocations that you can use as part of your preparation to heal (see page 48).

Step 2. Statement of Intent

Write out a statement of general intent for yourself as a healer and as a focus for your healing sessions (see page 49).

Step 3. Healing Sequences

Practice the healing sequences on pages 21, 35, and 38, but select some words from the list on page 57 as an aid to developing your awareness of what's happening and adjusting your input into the healing session.

For instance, you might select *agitated, cold,* and *resistant,* and endeavor to sense any instances of this in your patient's energy field. If you find an agitated area, practice calming or soothing it; warm a cold area and ease a resistant area into flow. Use your hands naturally and intuitively and hold an image of the changes you intend to make.

This chapter was written to help you think more deeply about the implications of being a healer, develop your healing perceptions and responses, and manage a healing session in detail. In the next chapter, we'll look at healing as a philosophy and process, and at the symbolic meaning of illness.

Chapter 4

The Meaning of Disease

*Finding our true selves—The symbolic meanings of symptoms—
Joshua's story—Exploring symptoms as symbols—Breakdown to
breakthrough—Chloe's story—Exercise*

The process of healing can be seen as a journey to new insight and maturity, rather than as a return to a state of health previously known. Disease and symptoms are communications from our bodies on behalf of the whole of our psyche or being. Learning and striving to be well stretches us physically, but also emotionally, mentally, and spiritually.

Illness has symbolic meaning. If the word *disease* is split, it becomes *dis-ease*. This is the state that often precedes illness and can be spiritual, emotional, physical, or mental in origin.

We should take seriously those times when we're uneasy in our lives or bodies. The expectations imposed on us, both by others and by ourselves, may cause us stress. The tendency is to give ourselves a good talking to, take a deep breath, call on our willpower, and then carry on with the same old patterns. We too easily forget that such dis-ease can eventually produce more chronic ill health and sickness.

"Mind over matter" is an attitude to life that's often greatly admired but frequently misunderstood. We endeavor to subjugate body and emotions to the discipline and direction of our minds. We are conditioned to, or filled with, expectations of what we ought to be. Parents, teachers, and society have an investment in molding or forcing us into conformity. We are pressured into pursuing interests seen by others as good for us. We must perform to a preset standard and generally become happy, normal, or well adjusted. Our minds learn to believe that these norms or expectations are right. We may turn ourselves inside out to please others and fulfil their ambitions for us. We desperately yearn for approval.

FINDING OUR TRUE SELVES

A gardener who decides to plant some unlabeled but interesting-looking seeds will watch their growth carefully, assessing their needs as they grow. He will be interested to observe their progress and see what sort of plant each is becoming. Should there be flower or fruit, he'll be delighted with the result. Whatever the shape, color, or size, he'll be content if each plant is healthy and flourishing. He'll let those that want to grow tall have support. He'll see that the shorter, bushier ones have enough light and ground space.

A gardener knows that a seed holds a certain blueprint or potential. It is useless to plant a tomato seed if you want to grow an oak tree; no amount of persuasion, tending, discipline, or threat will make the seed change. If the conditions are not right for the seed, it will sicken and die.

Of course, the analogy between a seed and a human being can be pushed too far, but nevertheless it serves to set us thinking about the nature of disease. However much we may struggle to gain approval and to be what others ask of us, our feelings and emotions will eventually make it clear if we're a square peg in a round hole.

If feelings are ignored and the mind pushes us on, or entrenches us further in areas where we cannot express the true self, the body will begin to collude. It will become the servant of our emotions because when the body fails, life change may be forced upon us. When we learn to listen both to our emotions and to our bodies, and understand the messages we are being given, then we may be able to choose change before change chooses us.

It's more difficult to avoid the signals of the body than of the mind. If the body's ill, we cannot continue. If we ignore the messages of minor symptoms, they may develop into something major, or we may have an accident.

Pain is an example. It's nature's way of signaling that something is wrong. If we merely kill the pain with pills in order to carry on our lifestyle without interruption, we may be choosing to ignore an important message and be in danger of leaving the real meaning behind the cause of our trouble undetected and untreated. If we don't examine our life pattern, a serious illness or breakdown may develop. Recurring headaches can develop into heart attacks or strokes. Life-threatening illnesses, forcing us to consider our quality of life, can develop from symptoms we choose to ignore.

Even when we attend to our symptoms, getting rid of them is not necessarily the way to true, whole health. To heal ourselves deeply, rather than merely being satisfied with removing symptoms, we may need to understand what they are telling us and be prepared to make such life changes as allow the true self to shine through. If we listen to symptoms in depth and at an early stage, we may not need to become seriously ill in order to shift the pattern. Symptoms can be ambassadors on behalf of our emotions and our true selves.

THE SYMBOLIC MEANINGS OF SYMPTOMS

Instead of seeing disease as an attacker or a monster, we should consider the symbolic wisdom that it encompasses. Symptoms certainly carry warnings in the early stages. They are potential friends or allies, and every symptom bears a different message. Although there may be a common thread in the message carried by a particular group of symptoms, the total communication to the individual manifesting such symptoms is unique and personal.

Lists suggesting symbolic meanings for symptoms should be used only as a guide to further personal insight. Many books give blanket indications of what dis-ease means for an individual, of emotional sources of dis-ease. Such information can be misleading, since the sources of dis-ease can vary from person to person—for instance, while breast cancer may often indicate an overattachment to family, this is not necessarily the case.

To be told that trouble with your gall bladder means you are unconsciously bitter may bring insight to some, but guilt and self-recrimination to others. As healers who may discuss the symbolic meaning of disease with our patients, we must take great care not to add a burden of guilt to the already existing burden of illness.

Bitterness (because of the gall) must certainly be considered by those with weakness in this area, but it is possible to open the exploration more gently. A less accusatory, categorical or judgmental approach would be to ask: "What is the bitter pill that life has presented me and caused me to swallow? Must I continue to swallow it? Are there any life or attitudinal changes I might make that would be to my advantage?"

There is an attitude to self-responsibility in alternative and complementary medicine circles that can all too easily add the burden of guilt to that of disease. Interpreting illness symbolically should not be a way of saying, "It's really all your fault. You've done this to yourself, so what are you going to do about it now?" Rather, the exploration of symptoms as symbols should be exciting, a piece of detective work enabling each symbol to be explored as a key to greater knowledge of how the potential of the true self might be discovered and released.

An exploration of the exact expression of the many symptoms that we, as humans, can manifest is beyond the scope of this book. But we can learn how to listen to symptoms as symbols and so aid our healing process. The points to remember are:

1. Disease and symptoms can be allies rather than enemies, telling us to look at our lifestyles and to perhaps open up more. As such, they can be a path for learning and self-empowerment. See also page 74.
2. There is often a greater wisdom within the sick self than in the conditioned well self.
3. Symptoms are signals from the sick self that all is not well, not only physically but emotionally and perhaps spiritually too.

It behooves us to look further at the concept of the parts of ourselves that manifest as conditioned well self, sick self, and true well self.

The Conditioned Well Self

Our longing for approval is one of the strongest of human urges. It places a powerful weapon in the hands of those who wield authority. The child's longing for approval invests parents and teachers with the power to fashion the basic mores and social graces that enable family and community life to run smoothly. This is necessary. All can be well if that authority is tempered with wisdom and love, but that same longing for approval can create a power that is subtly corrupt. Much can go wrong if love is possessive or when there is a chain reaction of conformity based on fear, when the requirements of society have not been questioned, or when a sense of frustration causes tunnel vision.

The psychologist Carl Rogers insisted that a major requirement for successful psychotherapy is that the therapist should be able to maintain an "unconditional positive regard" for the patient. This doesn't mean that the patient will not be helped toward behavioral changes or discernment, but that the basic human essence must be seen and valued before healthy growth can take place. Many parents and teachers would do well to remember and observe that axiom.

All too often the child gets a message of conditional love or regard. It's as if their parents are saying, "Do what we want you to do, become what we want you to become, be the success I never was, do not question our values, make us proud of you on our terms and all will be well, for after all we only want what's best for you—and having lived longer we know what's best for you."

This last phrase is undoubtedly reiterated with great sincerity. It should not, however, be an excuse for that lack of sensitivity that forces a developing being into an incompatible mold. Humility and insight both allow and positively support a freer choice.

These and similar influences lead us to acquire a conditioned well self, which is not our true self. We sense that in some way we're gaining approval. We've chosen the right job, we've made a "good" marriage, we've worked toward a lovely home, lots of material possessions, and the traditional 2.4 children. Conversely, we may feel that we're approved of because we've rejected all these values and are suitably scruffy, ill-fed, rebellious, and unemployed. Peer groups take over from parents as the approving authorities, and parents can project their own rebellions as well as their own conformities onto their children. In short, we only escape the conditioned well self when we take the courage to choose for ourselves.

The Sick Self

The conditioned well self easily gives rise to the sick self, leading us to pursue false values and false means of gaining self-respect. Too much conformity to the conditioned well self can lead us into mental, physical, emotional, or spiritual illnesses and breakdowns. Often, such breakdowns contain wisdom and force a reassessment of our lifestyle, life values, and choices. Although such hiatuses are devastating, break down of the conditioned well self into the sick self can be a means of breaking through to the true self.

Obviously, it is altogether better if we can reassess the patterns when we're in a state of un-ease or dis-ease rather than having to enter full sickness or breakdown to gain awareness. Pursuing insight is not always straightforward. There are ties that bind us to negative patterns and permissions we lack that can be very powerful inhibitors indeed. Releasing the conditioned well self to move on to who we truly are can be a scary business. When some "befriending" of the sick self takes place we may be amazed at the wisdom underlying the apparent obstacles it has thrown across our life path.

We get job-weary, bored, irritable, inexplicably overtired, or lose our sense of meaning. At such times, we force ourselves on because we see no way of releasing conditioned values and expectations. If we force too far, the sick self with its intrinsic underlying wisdom may step in. It's worth our while to learn to understand its language.

The True Well Self

We cannot overturn all the conditioned choices we've made—and will rarely want to. However, constant reassessment and attention to the things that truly make our hearts sing are important to the well-being and nourishment of the true well self. When this blossoms, vitality, energy, and posi- tive all-around healthfulness are released into our lives. To enable this, we have to be more aware of the compromises we've made and be open to modifying those that no longer work for us. When the true well self is honored, we follow the light and purpose of our higher selves with joy as easily and naturally as a sunflower's face follows the sun.

An approach to healing that endeavors to understand the wisdom of illness can lead us to see that there is a potent natural force within each of us that urges us to release a unique and powerful potential and to transform disease into true health. Thus, disease, more broadly understood, leads us to consider our natural blueprint. It does not only have to be an obstacle on our way through life, but a guide to self- realization.

It may seem strange to suggest that illness has benefits, yet it can be a means to getting things we lack in life, particularly before it reaches a chronic stage. As we begin to ask questions about the dynamics within illness, complex but interesting life stories emerge from the exploration. Joshua's story is an illustration of how deep the benefits of illness may lie.

JOSHUA'S STORY

Joshua came to me several times one winter for healing for sinus problems that followed the very frequent colds he was catching. Healing always seemed to help but did not prevent the problem from recurring. He worked in an office where there was air-conditioning. This meant that windows were rarely opened, and if one person caught a cold it invariably spread. Yet as the common cold season progressed, most of the others with whom Joshua worked seemed to develop some degree of immunity and were certainly not falling prey to each and every cold brought in by visitors or staff from other departments. It seemed to Joshua that someone only had to sniff, let alone sneeze, and he would be in for the familiar syndrome: an acute cold, followed by blocked sinuses. After the first day of a cold he would usually return to work, but once the sinuses became painful he had to take time off. His work was stressful, with deadlines to meet, and having to take days off increased his problems.

When Joshua asked me to help him explore whether there were underlying reasons locking him into this miserable and recurring pattern, I asked him whether he felt there were any benefits to his illness. He resisted this suggestion fairly strenuously. There were no benefits, he said, in having to take time off, miss important deadlines, build up a sickness record, and suffer the recurring misery of sinus pain. Despite the stress, Joshua liked his work and would far rather meet his deadlines than spend time at home with a blocked nose and throbbing sinuses. The unwanted time off was causing him more stress at work, and he didn't see it as an unconscious desire to take time out.

Obviously we had to go deeper, so we explored what else was going on in Joshua's life and how his being ill affected his household. He had been married to Faith for three years and said that they both described their relationship as "an inspiration." They met when Faith came to do some temping in Joshua's office. After graduating from high school, she took a year off and decided to train as a teacher. But then she contracted a very bad case of glandular fever. She missed most of a year of teachers' college and decided to delay any decision about whether and when she'd complete her training. Once she felt better, she traveled abroad with a group of friends, doing casual work here and there when funds got low. On returning to England, she signed on with a temp agency and met Joshua when she came to work at his office.

Joshua's childhood had not been easy. His mother died when he was quite young, and his father had been unable to

cope with looking after him. This meant that he was brought
up by relatives but, rather than staying with one family, was
shunted around between grandparents, aunts, and uncles.
His father maintained as much contact as possible, and
Joshua knew he cared. Although the relatives had all been
kind, real mothering was something that was suddenly cut
off from his life.

Faith enjoyed homemaking and was good at it. Her
temping meant that she could work hours that allowed her
to give full attention to Joshua. The comfort and together-
ness he enjoyed now that he was married were very precious
and healing to him. He and Faith wanted a few years
together before starting a family, and Faith toyed with the
idea of completing her lapsed teacher training so that she
could have the sort of career that blends most easily with
family responsibilities. Just before the onset of Joshua's recurring sinus problems, she applied to and was accepted at the
local college.

Although Joshua applauded this in principle and wanted
to support her education, it seemed that there were mixed
feelings in practice. Joshua knew that there would be a
disruption to the comfortable routine he now enjoyed when
college hours and the necessary study made their extra
demands on Faith.

As a child, Joshua remembered the times when he'd been
ill as times of comfort. Someone would always rise to the
occasion and give him the extra attention he craved. Faith,
worried about this bout of ill health that Joshua was having,
intimated that she might need to put off her return to college
to look after him and support him until he was better.

As Joshua spoke of all this, it was as though a light bulb
flashed for him and he could see that part of him was really
looking to Faith to mother him. He'd never ask her to delay
or forego something he knew she wanted to do for so long
and which was part of their joint plan for the future, but his

ill health made her offer the very thing he subconsciously wanted and gave him permission to consider accepting it.

When healing Joshua, I sensed a tightness in his heart chakra. Since colds are often more associated with the sacral and throat chakras, I wondered about this energetic symptom. Now it was explained. His marriage had opened his heart but he was still very vulnerable from his childhood. His inner child felt threatened by the new phase that Faith's return to college would bring about.

Since one of the standard symbolic meanings for sinus problems can be repressed or unshed tears, I asked Joshua how much he had been able to mourn for his mother. He said that one of his aunts had suggested to him that he should stay strong for his father since his father was staying strong for him and had discouraged his natural tears and sadness. He had earned a lot of family compliments for being "brave," but now the imminent disruption of the status quo was tapping into old material. He didn't feel able to ask Faith to go on mothering him—but part of him was not dealing with the potential loss of this aspect very well.

As Joshua's understanding of the emotional issues underlying this bout of sinus infections increased, he went for some counseling sessions to help heal his inner child and release the blocked grief. When Faith understood what was happening, she found a creative compromise. She wanted to complete her training as quickly as possible, but there was an option available to do it less intensively over a longer period and she happily agreed to change to this more relaxed schedule.

The sinus problems soon began to lessen, both in frequency and intensity. Joshua continued to come for healing, to help with the process that was going on in his counseling, but he was now set up to go from strength to strength.

This all took place some years ago. Faith completed her teaching degree and taught for a while, until they decided to start a family. Now they have two growing children. They keep in touch with me from time to time. Joshua loves family life and Faith is doing some substitute teaching with no plans to go permanent or full time. On every level they have reached a creative compromise, are able to support each other, and understand the dynamics of their relationship more deeply.

EXPLORING SYMPTOMS AS SYMBOLS

Interpreting symptoms as symbols helps us uncover layer after layer as we seek to understand the deep wisdom within disease. Our bodies speak a very simple, even primitive language. We derive the most from symbols when we live alongside them for a while, rather than rushing to interpret them intellectually. Symbols are rich and many-faceted, yet in another sense economical, since so much comes out of apparent simplicity. Recognizing that a symbol exists starts a communication process with it, and within ourselves.

Most of us find ourselves, at some time in our lives, in a situation where we recognize that we are not totally content. We are working too many hours in a job we do not really enjoy or that stretches us too much or not enough; we live in a town when we would rather be in the country, or vice versa; we cannot understand why those things we have always worked toward no longer seem right or comfortable.

We make excuses to delay making changes or rationalizing our lifestyles. The present job must continue because it enables the children to have a better education. We are used to two holidays a year. Yes, we have a huge mortgage, but it provides us with a lovely home. If I work hard now and put up with stressful conditions, I'll be able to retire early. If I make changes, I might not like the new life any better than the present one. The sacrifices I'm making now are benefiting others, and if I make changes they might feel let down. I fear choice itself. It would be selfish to change. It's too late to train or retrain. Others might be disappointed in me if I say how unhappy I am.

In areas where we have been heavily conditioned by parents, society, or circumstances to strive for a certain lifestyle or to achieve certain standards, our minds try to exert willpower over emotion and even over matter. Our emotions help us question the old order. They encourage us to find and live our own personal truths and values, and to get that vital glimpse of our true selves. The body interacts and colludes with the emotions, and produces symptoms that make us take notice of the fact that all is not well.

Eventually, if the symptoms are pressing enough, we may be forced into a life change. The Monday headache appears every weekday; we have no energy to enjoy our leisure time on the weekend and so spend it in sleep or depression; a medical check warns us about blood pressure. If we take no notice of the early warnings, the daily headache can escalate into heart attack or stroke, the weekend depression results in our finding signs of impending serious illness.

The dramatic and life-threatening illnesses ask us, "Do you want to live or die?" Our minds and conditioning can weld us to lifestyles that sustain life but are not about living as our true selves would have us live. In such circumstances, the vital spark within us may be more dead than alive.

In serious illness it is more than the actual symptoms themselves that court the possibility of death. Often those symptoms have only come about because our souls are weary and our spiritual vitality and purpose have been lost. Part of our recovery will be to rekindle the spark and to revise our life choices so that it burns brightly once more.

That inner spark might be called joy. It produces joy and is fed by joy. Lives that become joyless are lives where illness may issue its underlying challenge. We describe serious illnesses as life-threatening, but symbolically they might also be seen as life-seeking. They threaten the status quo but may force the changes our true selves require to live at all.

BREAKDOWN TO BREAKTHROUGH

The annals of healing have many stories to tell of people struck down by serious illness or accident, and of the wondrous recoveries they make when their lifestyles are revised. One client discovered an aggressive cancer lump in her breast. As she recovered physically from the even more aggressive treatment required, she decided to go on the adventures in life she had always been putting on hold. Part of the buildup to her illness had been the loss of a partner. Now she realized that she could, if she so chose, be free.

She sold her assets and found simple accommodation in a warm land of her choice. Gradually, she allowed herself only to make those choices that made her heart sing. In time, she met and married a new partner, and her present life choices come from a different place within her being than did her earlier ones. She is fit, well, and full of joy. She is more healthy in body, mind, and spirit than she had ever thought it possible to be. Her true self lives.

Another client, following in the family tradition of farming, became seriously affected by hay fever and allergic asthma. He suddenly revealed a heart's dream to live in town and run a good restaurant. After retraining, he was able to do this, and now he has no allergic symptoms, even when he visits the family farm or gives a hand with some of the old jobs. He works hard for his dream, but his life spark has been reignited.

The body does not become ill without reason. Most of us have constitutionally vulnerable areas and produce certain types of symptoms. Although familiar, these may well be urging us gradually toward major life changes, or to more simple ones based on life issues we are not fully addressing but which are affecting us more than we realize. Some of the language we use about life and relationships gives us initial clues to understanding the symbolic deeper layers of our symbols:

- I can't stomach it any more. It turns my stomach. I'm having a gut reaction. It sticks in my throat. I'm sick of it.
- My heart is heavy. I'm sick at heart. My heart aches.
- I feel as though I have the weight of the world on my shoulders. I feel so stiff-necked. My life is rigid. It's a pain in the butt.
- I am world weary. It's doing my head in. It's getting me down.
- It irritates me. It makes me shudder. It makes me want to burst. It's a prickly/sticky situation.
- All is not well.

Such phrases are descriptive of our un-ease or dis-ease on a physical, emotional, mental, and spiritual level. They describe how certain things in life can affect us and what they can do to us. As we express things in such a way, we may hear ourselves and decide that the way things are is not good enough, and we must take steps to resolve a situation. If we listen to what we're saying about ourselves and, as a result, act to change or improve things, then the actual pain in the back, sickness, or stiff neck may not manifest physically. Our language is a warning. On the other hand, if we endure too much the body can react.

Judy, a client of mine, knew that her back and neck were her most vulnerable areas. She was in a job where recent cuts had made the work she once loved very frustrating. Her marriage was going through a tricky patch and her twins, a boy and girl aged nineteen years, were in the process of leaving home for a year before entering college. Everything familiar was in a process of change and falling away. When she came with a really sore back and very stiff neck that were resistant to osteopathic treatment, we worked out the following list of questions for her to ask herself:

- Am I being stiff-necked about something?
- Could I gain from being *more* stiff-necked about something? (i.e., is my body doing it for me?)
- Is something (or someone!) being a pain in the neck to me?
- Am I being a pain in the neck to myself or someone else?
- Am I sticking my neck out unnecessarily about some matter?
- Should I stick my neck out more in the present situation?
- Am I being too rigid?
- Am I being too flexible?
- Is someone on my back?
- Am I on someone else's back?
- Am I carrying too much for myself and/or others?
- Am I carrying enough? Taking enough responsibility?

Each question needs to be reversed (as above), and in the end the person exhibiting the symptoms is the only one who can give the answers. What one person experiences as stress, another may feel as positive challenge. In looking at the lives of others, we may judge them to be under a particular pressure, but they themselves may not feel this to be so. In using symptoms as symbols to help us to see the wisdom in disease, we need to be in touch with what we feel about certain situations, rather than what we think of them.

As it was, Judy said that she could answer almost all these questions affirmatively. Work, marriage, and children were all weighing on her and she on them. At one moment she would be too rigid or stiff-necked, at the next too flexible. She was carrying a great deal for others but, in a sense, not enough for herself. She realized that she hadn't given sufficient thought to what she really wanted as the outcome of this period of change. How would she like her own quality of living to be when she came through the various areas of transition that life was currently presenting her with?

Judy considered this and began to set some new boundaries at home and at work. She couldn't make immediate life changes at that point, but there were various ways in which she could ease the burden on herself. She began to see that there was opportunity as well as difficulty in whatever lay ahead, and that she could negotiate for a positive outcome to the changes that had been thrust upon her. She could take things more lightly, not feel so burdened, and see hope, rather than imminent disaster, ahead.

A couple of years ago, I caught a virus that left my body, particularly my legs, full of aches and pains. I lost ease of movement and had to do everything much more slowly. I had known for some time that I was living at a very hectic pace, sometimes forcing myself to keep it up. My body was asking me to slow down. I interpreted this as quite a serious warning and have since tried to rest more, have more fun, look after my body, take more space for myself, and get some of my commitments into proportion.

Looking at the language of symptoms and how we speak of life and its effects leads us to the first layers of understanding symptom as symbol. But there are even deeper areas that the symptoms our bodies produce can tell us about. Understanding symbolic body messages can result in an exploration of bodily memory and its links with our emotions. It can guide us to excise deep wounds that have been buried in the profound recesses of our beings. The body often aims to keep a flow going between unconscious and conscious, particularly where emotions and matters relating to the blossoming of the true self are concerned.

Healing our total being, taking spiritual, mental, and

emotional aspects into account in addition to the physical, necessitates the courage to be honest with ourselves and to gain deeper self-knowledge. It means seeking a deeper understanding of our interactions with the world, with relationships, and with all interpersonal communication. More than this, it means learning about our intricate intrapersonal communications and the dynamics of our complex beings. Although some of these explanations are of a self-healing nature, it can be within the scope of the healer to encourage patients to make such explorations for themselves as part of the healing process.

I have quoted the following case history in my book *Chakras—A New Approach to Healing Your Life,* but it shows clearly some of the deeper causes that are held within the causality of some of our ills.

CHLOE'S STORY

Chloe, an Afro-Caribbean client whose family came to live in southern England before she was one year old, wanted to explore the deeper cause of a pulled ankle tendon. The original injury had occurred two years previously while she and her partner were leading a group into a dance at a social gathering. The continuing pain, stiffness, and weakness in her ankle were still resistant to improvement. She had explored the possibilities that she was carrying too much on behalf of others, or not being true to her inner self.

This line of questioning revealed some valuable insights, and Chloe had taken steps to make changes and redress certain balances, yet her ankle still did not heal. Medical investigation simply confirmed that the tendons had been sprained and were still weak. There was no other physical injury or apparent physical contributing cause.

Chloe's right ankle was the one affected. The right side of the body is symbolically associated with those aspects of life

demanding qualities of focus, direction, thrusting, activity—
the masculine principle or yang energy. The left side connects
with the areas of life asking for qualities of diffuse awareness,
subtlety, yielding, receptivity—the feminine principle or yin
energy.

Bearing this in mind, I asked Chloe whether she most
often put her right, masculine, yang, leadership side forward in life, or whether she tended to function more from
her feminine, yielding, receptive side?

Chloe felt that life had pushed her toward being "up
front," "in the lead" and "visible." She was an attractive
woman in a good relationship but felt that in many ways the
development of her truly feminine side had taken a back seat.

Chloe's family had always pushed her to do well at school.
In art classes she discovered a talent for design but had
never been allowed to enjoy it in a relaxed way. Her gift was
taken seriously, and she'd been expected to work hard and
get top grades and a degree. She thoroughly enjoyed her
present job, working with a design and display team for a
large organization, yet she often had a sense of frustration
and felt that her talent was always too developed and
focused. She was never able to indulge in it for its own sake
or to dabble with all the potentials that could have been open
to her.

Remarking that the injury to her ankle occurred when she
was leading others into a dance, I asked her to consider
whether her right ankle might be telling her that the masculine side needed a rest and that it could be time to give the
left, feminine side more chance to develop. She felt that this
explanation was too simplistic and that there was something
deeper and more complex involved.

I asked Chloe to close her eyes and see what image came
to mind when she considered her right ankle and its injury.
After a while she said she could see herself, aged about seven
years old, in a Brownie uniform. The word *tenderfoot* accom-
panied this image. When asked to associate the word and the

image, Chloe began to talk about a phase in her life that she had not remembered so clearly before.

As a tenderfoot Brownie, working toward full enrollment to receive the Brownie badge and become a full Brownie member, Chloe was required to do at least one good turn every day. To keep a check on this, the troop leader gave each of the tenderfoot Brownies a card and some stick-on stars. As a good turn was done, a star would be stuck on the card. This was the equivalent of earning Brownie points. At the end of each week, before the Brownie meeting, Chloe had to get one of her parents to sign the card to verify the number of good turns completed that week.

Chloe's parents had always required her to share tasks in the household. They told her that any good turn for her Brownie membership had to be something over and above the things she was normally expected to do. Since quite a lot was already demanded of her, especially given her young age, she had difficulty in finding something extra each day that her parents would agree to mark on her card as her good turn. Indeed, if she didn't do one of her usual chores to perfection, even the extra good turn was not considered worthy of a star.

At the next Brownie meeting, Chloe had the least number of good turns on her record. She knew that her friends did not help in the home nearly as much as she did and was desperately upset when the troop leader told her that she obviously needed to try harder if she truly wanted to be an enrolled Brownie. She was unable to explain to her parents what was happening. They consistently refused to consider anything within their normal high demands of her as a good turn. Eventually, in desperation and although it cut her off from many of her friends, Chloe gave up Brownies and the tenderfoot requirements. Her parents then criticized her for lack of commitment and consistency.

As this painful memory surfaced, Chloe realized that there

were similar factors operating in her current situation. Although she loved her work, knew she was good at it, and often willingly worked unpaid overtime, she was continually being overlooked or under-rewarded when it came to promotions and raises. She recognized that she tended not to fight this particular circumstance.

As a black woman in a white culture, Chloe had learned the value of self-assertion, but she now saw that she didn't expect to be paid or rewarded for her dedication. She felt she had to be more than exceptional before recognition could come her way. She was doing more than others in the team but not getting her Brownie points.

In relation to her foot, Chloe had the insight that she was often putting her "best foot forward" to the point of stress, without receiving her just reward or support. Her physical foot had been showing her that something else was lacking and that an old pattern needed to be recognized and dealt with. She needed more balance between right and left, yin and yang. She needed to use her yang side to make sure that she was fairly treated. An underlying resentment was beginning to surface that might affect her decisions about, and attitudes toward, her work.

A few weeks later, she reported that she'd requested, and was awarded, a long overdue promotion and salary increase. Her right foot was much less painful and she felt that it was healing successfully at last. We'd gotten to the root cause of the continuing tender foot.

The following exercises are based on the ideas in this chapter. Do them for yourself—it's always good for healers to check their own well-being from time to time. Having applied them to your own life, you might feel confident enough to help someone else begin to understand and explore the deeper meanings of sickness and symptoms.

Exercise
Analyzing Illness

Look back to page 76 and the section entitled "Breakdown to Breakthrough." This looks at some of the language of life and illness, and moves on to mention Judy and the exploration she made that helped her back improve. With pen and paper at hand, use this section to help you make the following two explorations:

1. Think of a situation in your present life that you're aware is not in balance or is irking you in some way. Reflect on it as meditatively as possible. Be aware of any feelings that arise and of any bodily sensations that might accompany these feelings.

- Write down single, simple sentences that describe what this situation does to you when it has to be dealt with. You might write phrases such as: It stifles me, It irritates me, or It makes me feel sick.
- When you've written all you need to, reflect on the words and phrases on your paper. Highlight some of them in color—especially any that are not only ways of expressing how you feel about the situation but may actually have converted, even if only mildly, into bodily sensations or symptoms.
- Think about any actual or attitudinal changes you might be able to make that will help you handle the situation better next time. Do you need to ask for help and support from others when perhaps you've been struggling with this situation alone?

2. Refer back to the sections beginning on page 67 about the conditioned well self, the sick self, and the true well self.

Think about these and try to sense how they manifest in your own life and attitudes.

- Take three separate sheets of paper or make three divisions on a larger sheet, and then draw your conditioned well self, your sick self and your true well self. Note the posture each takes up and the colors you choose for them. (Matchstick drawings are fine if you're not artistic.)
- Draw a balloon (as in a word comic strip) coming from the mouth of each of these selves. After reflection and sensing into the nature of each, write in the balloon the words that you feel each of these aspects might want to say to you right now. Is there any action or adjustment you might need to make in your life as a result of bringing these words to awareness?

Our spiritual, mental, emotional, and physical selves don't exist on separate islands. They're in constant interaction and communication, often striving to find balance through a process of which we're usually only peripherally aware. We have to take notice of our bodies to achieve the mechanics of living. Thus our bodies bring to the surface those areas that require our attention. These are deeper than the physical symptoms that manifest as dis-ease.

Deep healing requires us to assist our patients in listening to the wise messages the sick self can hold, to modify the pull of the conditioned well self, and to make space for their true selves to blossom and flourish. The next chapter looks at the ways we can develop an awareness of the subtle bodies' colors to help us assist patients in the search for health and vitality.

Chapter 5

Color Healing

The chakras and colors—How chakras link to life and health—
Associating illness with the chakras—More about colors and their
qualities—Seeing, sensing, and perceiving—Exercises

In considering the work of healers and of healing intervention, the idea that we work mainly with the subtle
energy field, or aura, around us is central to this book. A
basic understanding of this concept gives us enough knowledge of the chakras to be able to use these energy centers
as areas of focus when healing with our hands. This knowledge, in turn, brings a structured approach to healing
intervention. As we saw in Chapter 3, knowing a little more
can help, both by providing a language with which to
interpret healing sensations and by firming up our inner
statements of healing intent. In this chapter, we explore
the ways that increasing our awareness of color can help
our understanding of healing energies.

We can heal on a sentient level and/or visually. Many
healers see colors quite naturally when healing. Color
knowledge helps visual healing, but also means that the
nonvisual healer can impart colors mentally during a

healing session, for example by *thinking* "clear blue to the throat chakra."

THE CHAKRAS AND COLORS

The illustration on page 90 shows the positions and names of the chakras (see also page 31). The seven major chakras—crown, brow, throat, heart, solar plexus, sacral, and root—are linked to the seven colors of the rainbow spectrum: violet for the crown, indigo for the brow, blue for the throat, green for the heart, yellow for the solar plexus, orange for the sacral, and red for the root.

Each chakra is responsible for producing its spectrum color to feed into the physical body and the auric field in order to keep the whole being healthy on every level. The alter major chakra, though important to the chakra system, is technically a minor chakra, and its colors deviate from the normal rainbow sequence (see page 94).

The healthy being is a radiant, rainbow being. Part of healing intervention is to detect where this rainbow radiance may be faltering and to channel healing energy so that a subtle luminosity is restored. When our subtle energies are radiantly full of luminosity and rainbow color, this penetrates through to body, mind, spirit, and emotions, and manifests in vitality for life.

In conditions of tiredness, emotional upset, or the onset of physical illness, the chakras benefit by being fed, each with its own color. This feeding can occur through the hands and intent of a healer, through visualization, with the aid of colored lights or transparencies, and with the use of crystals.

Although each chakra needs its home spectrum color and is responsible for the production of that color for the whole auric field, the root chakra is not only red, the solar plexus not just yellow, and so on. Each and every color may be present in each and every chakra, but if its home color is not also strong and flowing, then unease, imbalance, or disease exists within the total being. This may be transitory, since our auras, chakras, and colors change many times during a day and also when we sleep.

When a healer holds their hands over the chakra energy points, the flow of healing helps to energize and balance the chakra, and restore and harmonize the colors in the chakras and in the aura. The healer does not have to be thinking of color for this to happen. If balance is present or being brought about in the chakra through the giving of healing, then it turns, vibrates, and is full of light. It produces its own color in a balanced shade and in correct amounts to blend with all other chakra colors, energize the auric field, and produce radiant, rainbow energy for life.

Although simple direction of healing with the hands has an effect on the colors within the chakras, the healing procedure becomes more specific if the healer also visualizes color, with directed color being used to feed and balance active or underactive chakras. Some healers quite naturally and clearly see or sense what is happening with chakras, colors, and auric energies. When the chakra is sensed as lifeless, its colors and other colors in the aura may be seen or sensed as weak or pale. If the chakra is over-energized, the colors may be too intense.

Healthy chakra and auric colors look like stained glass when sunlight passes through it: fairly intense, bright, and translucent. When there is imbalance in us, our colors may be opaque, ethereal, or faint. We may have a great deal of one color and little of another. Because colors are also related to gifts and abilities, it's natural to have more of some than of others, but when one color is struggling to maintain itself or is almost totally absent and another color is too prominent, all is not well.

In the healing exercises suggested in this book, much attention is given to the chakra points. This is because at these points the state of health can be sensed, and also because—

if the chakras are healed, balanced, and energized—the self-healing mechanism can be reactivated and helped to work smoothly.

At energy interchange points, the chakras are affected by our emotions, thoughts, and reactions to and interaction with our environment. They are responsible for producing and regulating color in our auric field. The state of our chakras affects the health of our total being, while the state of our total health can be read from the qualities and distribution of our chakric energies and colors.

Chakras have petals and stems, with an energy flow from petals to stems that incorporates a subtle blending and elimination system. The stems open to let unwanted energy out, and the petals open, pulse, and rotate in response to life situations of all kinds. When life saddens, angers, excites, or moves us, as well as when we're in different states of physical health, our chakras respond. The quality and distribution of their colors will change as they endeavor to keep us balanced and well. When things are severely out of equilibrium, the chakras may lose vitality and need special help if they're to go on doing their part in keeping us physically, mentally, emotionally, and spiritually healthy.

Any color can be present in any chakra, but the truly healthy chakra must also produce its own color note very strongly. The distribution and quality of colors in the chakras not only give information about our health at the moment but, when perceived or read clairvoyantly, can help in knowing where our innate strengths and weaknesses lie.

How Chakras Link to Life and Health

Chakras are linked not only to color but also to key words, developmental stages, elements, senses, to each of the seven "bodies" in our auric field, to glands and fragrances, and to crystals or gemstones. (Suggestions for using crystals and

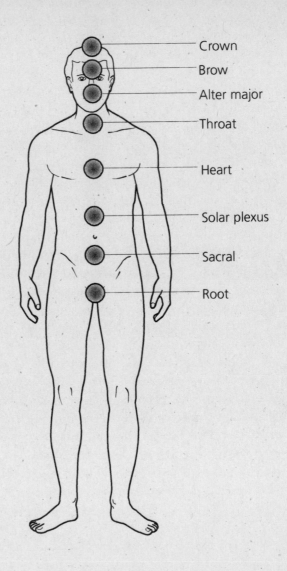

Crown
Brow
Alter major
Throat
Heart
Solar plexus
Sacral
Root

The positions and names of the most important chakras.

fragrances for healing are given in Chapter 7.) Informing ourselves about these connections will gradually strengthen the basis of knowledge from which we can work as healers.

Root Chakra

The root chakra is located in the perineum, which is the area midway between the anus and the genitals. The petals face downward, between the legs, and the stem faces upwards into the central column. It is naturally and healthily slightly open. The key words are rootedness, incarnation, acceptance, preservation, and concept. It is linked to the developmental stage up to between three and five years, and to the main color of red and secondary colors of brown and mauve. Its element is earth. Its sense is smell. It is associated with the physical body and the gonad glands (testes in men and ovaries in women). At the root, the fragrances of cedarwood and patchouli quiet, while musk, lavender, and hyacinth stimulate. Its crystals are smoky quartz, garnet, alexandrite, ruby, agate, bloodstone, onyx, tiger's eye, and rose quartz.

Sacral Chakra

The sacral chakra is to be found approximately two fingers below the navel. The stem corresponds to the sacrum area in the spine. The key words are security, sense of others, sexuality, creativity, power, empowerment, cocreativity, and sincerity. It's connected with the developmental ages of three to five to eight years. Its main color is orange and the secondary colors are amber and gold. Its element is water, its sense taste. It is linked to the etheric body (see Chapter 6 for more information about the subtle bodies). The glandular connection is to the lymphatics. Its quieting fragrances are musk and amber, its stimulating ones are rosemary and rose geranium. Its crystals are amber, citrine, topaz, aventurine, moonstone, and jasper.

Solar Plexus Chakra

The solar plexus chakra is situated just below the sternum, extending down to the navel, and the stem is in the corresponding position at the back. The key words are logic, reason, opinion, assimilation, psychic intuition, and identity. Its developmental age link is from eight to twelve years. Its main color is yellow and the secondary colors are gold and rose. The element is fire, the sense sight, and the subtle body is the astral. The glandular connection is to the adrenals. The quieting fragrances are vetivert and rose, with bergamot and ylang-ylang as stimulants. The solar plexus crystals are yellow citrine, apatite, calcite, kunzite, rose quartz, iron pyrites (fools' gold), yellow topaz, and malachite.

Heart Chakra

The heart chakra is located on the same level as the physical heart but in the center of the body, with the stem at the back. The key words and phrases are compassion, feeling, tenderness, love and search for the divine, love of others, and detachment. The associated developmental age is from twelve to fifteen years, while its main color is spring green, with subsidiary colors of rose and rose amethyst. The element is air, the sense touch, and it is connected to the subtle body known as the feeling body.

The glandular link is to the thymus. (The functioning of some glands in the body remains something of a mystery. The thymus is one of these. It's part of the lymphatic system, situated directly below the thyroid and parathyroid glands. It secretes a hormone known as thymic humoral factor. Between the ages of twelve and fifteen in the maturing human, the thymus gland begins to reduce in size. It is thought to have a connection with growth and with the progression from childhood to adulthood.) The fragrances of sandalwood and rose are quieting to the heart while pine and honeysuckle are stimulating. The crystals for the heart are emerald, green calcite, amber, azurite, chrysoberyl, jade, and rose and watermelon tourmalines.

Throat Chakra

The throat chakra is located at the neck, with petals in front and a stem at the back. The key words are expression, responsibility, communication, and universal truth. The developmental age is between fifteen and twenty-one years. The main color is blue, the subsidiaries are silver and turquoise. The associated element is ether or akasha (see Glossary, page 188). The sense at the throat is hearing, the subtle body is the mental body, and the glandular connections are to the thyroid and parathyroids. The quieting fragrances are lavender and hyacinth. Patchouli and white musk stimulate the throat chakra. The gemstones are lapis lazuli, aquamarine, sodalite, turquoise, and sapphire.

Brow Chakra

The brow chakra is located above and between the eyes, with a stem at the back of the head. The key words are spirit, completeness, inspiration, insight, and command. The main color is indigo, with subsidiaries of turquoise and mauve. The element at the brow is radium and the subtle body link is to the higher mental. The gland is the pineal. The quieting fragrances are white musk and hyacinth, and the stimulating ones are violet and rose geranium. The crystals are amethyst, purple apatite, azurite, calcite, pearl, sapphire, and blue and white fluorite. (There is no associated developmental stage for the throat chakra.)

Crown Chakra

The crown chakra is situated at the top of the head, with petals facing upward and a stem going down into the central column. The key words are soul, surrender, release, and incoming will. The main color is violet, and white and gold are the subsidiary colors. The element as given by guides is magnetum, but this has not yet been discovered for inclusion in tables of elements. The subtle body link is to the soul, ketheric, or causal body, and the glandular connection is the pituitary. The quieting fragrances for the crown chakra are rosemary and bergamot, while violet and amber stimulate. The crystals are diamond, white tourmaline, jade, snowy quartz, and celestite.

Alter Major Chakra

The alter major chakra is located with its petals in the area of the nose. Its positive energy center is in its stem, situated where the back of the head begins to curve around into the neck. This location corresponds to the "old" or "lizard" brain before the division into right and left hemispheres. The key words are instinct, resonance, rhythm, duality, devic nature, and healing. The principal color is brown and the secondary colors are yellow ochre and olive green. The element is wet earth and the sense, shared with the root chakra, is smell. The subtle body link is to the instinctual and lower causal, with the same glandular connection to the adrenals as for the solar plexus. The quieting fragrances are musk and cedarwood, the stimulating ones violet and rose geranium. The crystals are carnelian, tiger's eye, snowflake obsidian, fossils, and peacock stone.

ASSOCIATING ILLNESS WITH THE CHAKRAS

When looking for the deeper and symbolic meaning held by symptoms and disease, appropriate associations can be made to the chakras. Making such connections will guide us as to where the healing might most appropriately be focused. For instance, Joshua (see page 70) needed healing for his heart chakra but also for his sacral, solar plexus, and root chakras. Life had closed his heart, and he had been emotionally

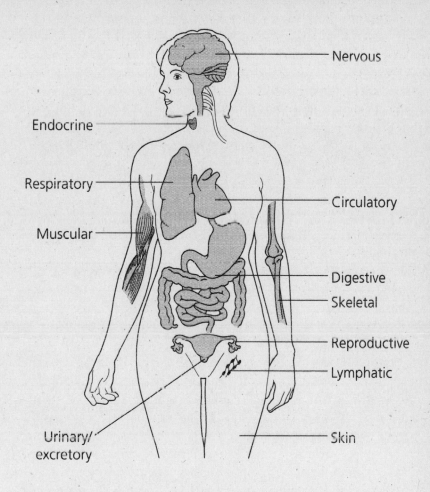

In a healthy person, the major systems of the body (shown simplistically above) act together in a coordinated way to ensure the smooth functioning of the body. Some systems, such as the muscular and skeletal, extend throughout the body, while the principal organs of others, like the digestive and reproductive, are more localized.

undernourished as a child (root chakra). His self-image and confidence in his own power was vulnerable (sacral and solar plexus). Giving healing to these chakras and teaching him to heal them himself helped his process of recovery.

My patient with aggressive breast cancer (see page 76) was always very controlled by her conditioned well self and was not able to follow her heart. She needed healing for her heart chakra, but also for her sacral chakra, which is associated with power and empowerment, her solar plexus, the identity center and fire energy chakra, and her throat chakra, to encourage her in true self-expression.

The farmer who had really always wanted to run a restaurant needed healing for his throat and sacral chakras to enable self-expression and empowerment, and also for his heart chakra because of his vulnerablility.

Judy (see page 77) needed strength in her solar plexus chakra to help her in finding her new identity, at her sacral chakra for courage to empower herself, at her throat chakra to help her self-expression, and at her alter major chakra to help her change in rhythm and pattern of life.

Chloe's (see page 80) root, sacral, heart, and throat chakras needed specific healing flow. She was loved but in many ways undernurtured, with heavy demands put on her. This affected her root chakra. The experience of over-rigid control by others made her sacral chakra rather tight, and the general conditions of her childhood gave her a painful vulnerability that could be helped by healing her heart chakra. Never having felt that she had permission to be her true self affected the flow and connection between her sacral and throat chakras.

Because chakra issues are complex, only a basic idea of their connections has been given here. As a healer, simply becoming familiar with these connections will support your intuitive approach to focusing your healing sessions and will help you understand why your intuition may draw you to certain areas. For more comprehensive information about chakras, refer to my books *Working with Your Chakras* and *Chakras—A New Approach to Healing Your Life*.

MORE ABOUT COLORS AND THEIR QUALITIES

As a nonprofessional healer, you will mostly use color thoughts, intentions, and visualizations as an extension to your natural, intuitive, energetic healing of the chakras, since these require no specific apparatus. Here's a little more information about colors and their qualities.

The different colors we see in our world are brought about by vibration and light. Each color has its own specific vibration, with red being the lowest on the scale and violet the highest. (Some shades of magenta may have a higher vibration than violet, which perhaps indicates that we are moving gradually toward being able to perceive a wider range of vibrations than has previously been possible.)

There are beneficial and antagonistic aspects of colors, usually defined by shade and tone. Softer, blending, or warm tones are beneficial. Harsh, garish, or muddy tones are antagonistic.

On the beneficial side: *red* is for warmth, life force, energy, passion, and celebration; *orange* is for vitality, initiation, creativity, and sexuality; *yellow* is for light, springtime, new beginnings, clarity, and joy; *green* is for growth, peace, rest fulness, and compassion; *blue* is for coolness, royalty, prayer, communication, and healing; *indigo* and *violet* are for richness, ritual, spirituality, and achievement.

On the antagonistic side: *red* is for danger, anger, wounding, and desecration; *orange* is for violence, aggression, negative power, and destruction; *yellow* is for criticism, cowardice, tawdriness, and loss of hope; *green* is for jealousy, bitterness, misfortune, and poisoning; *blue* is for coldness, cruelty, death, and deterioration; *indigo* and *violet* are for aloofness, misuse of power, and loss of hope.

Black is the absorption of all colors. Beneficially, it means dignity, mourning, the unknown, elegance, incubation, and containment. Antagonistically, it can signify evil, nightmare, rape, death, and the void. *White* is the reflection of all colors. Beneficially, it means innocence, virginity, freshness, neutrality, grace, and divinity. Antagonistically, it is blankness, harshness, shallowness, and cowardly surrender.

Silver and *gold* are the colors of the sun and moon. Traditionally, silver represents the feminine principle and gold the masculine. On the beneficial side, *silver* stands for cleansing, gentle strength, purity, natural rhythms, ebb and flow, mirroring, reflections, and vision. In its antagonistic aspect, it is coldness, harshness, rigidity, and treachery. Beneficially, *gold* is abundance, the divine, high spiritual attainment, warmth, harmony, and perfection. Antagonistically, it represents materialism, opulence, false values, and false images.

Pink in beneficial shades means love, tenderness, romance, birth, childlikeness, and fragrance. Antagonistically, it stands for faint-heartedness, childishness, lack of taste, and artificiality.

Brown has the beneficial attributes of fertility, containment, seed-time, harvest, and mellowness. Antagonistically, it represents blockage, filth, obstacles, depression, and despair.

Sometimes the difference between the beneficial and antagonistic side of a color is experienced in the shade or tone as suggested above. At other times the context in which the color is experienced will define whether its nature is beneficial or antagonistic. All meanings should be seen not as portents but as messages that help to bring clarity and choice.

Developing Awareness of Auric Color

As a healer, being able to see the colors and shades of a patient's aura is a great help in knowing what a patient needs and perhaps in making a deeper, symbolic diagnosis of what is not well. Some healers sense the colors and the quality each shade or tone carries without actually seeing them. Others say they can smell color and whether it is in positive or negative manifestation. It's possible gradually to come to know a color, tone, or shade by its energy—or simply an inner knowing (see "Sensing the Energy of Colors," page 101).

People who feel themselves drawn to healing and motivated to practice it often find that their sensitivities develop, and an increasing amount of subtle information floods in. You can struggle to develop color awareness or vision, but mostly it just happens with practice. You suddenly realize that you simply know such things as: this patient needs more yellow or more blue; this root chakra is not vibrating as well as it might because it needs feeding with a soft red; that patient is manifesting such a bright shade of orange in their spectrum that other colors are overwhelmed and the whole system is out of balance. Having a basic knowledge of and vocabulary about colors and chakras helps you express what you sense or perceive when you heal, so that more specific healing interventions emerge naturally.

If you want to be more aware of color in your healing and use colors more consciously and fluently in your healing intent, simply inform yourself about them and then relax until the day comes when you realize that they have become a natural part of your healing thinking and perception. You may or may not be actively seeing the colors by then, but you'll perceive them through your senses and sensitivity.

SEEING, SENSING, AND PERCEIVING

When dealing with subtle energies, colors, and the auric field, the whole question of sensing, seeing, and perception needs to be considered. I have found that many healers in

training hold themselves back or create an obstacle in the
development of their sensitivity by having an expectation
that the perception of subtle energies has to be an actual
seeing with the physical eyes. This is not so and, I believe, is
the actuality for only a very limited number of individuals.
Perception is much broader and more complex than physical seeing.

As sighted individuals, we take seeing our environment
for granted and may have minimal awareness of the other
complex ways in which we gather information about the
environment. Any blind person can tell us that a sightless
world is still a perceptual world. When physical sight is
denied, data floods in through other senses, which become
more sharpened.

The first exercise in this book (see page 14) was designed
to help you become more aware of the auric or energy field
that surrounds each one of us. We extend, energetically,
beyond our physical bodies. This energy field can be subtly
perceived or electrically sensed. Beyond that, the field itself
has sensate perception. We take in information through
seeing, hearing, touching, smelling, and tasting, but something else is added in our full perception that is more than
knowledge and experience, and is a part of the renowned
sixth sense. Not only is this something else added when all
our other senses are functioning, but it also exists when the
other senses are, for some reason, disabled, blocked, or muted.

If we sit quietly in a dark room, we can often sense
whether it is empty or furnished. This can happen even
without the clue of noise, which would tell us something by
the way it echoed or was absorbed. We can sense if there's
furniture or other objects because gradually the space taken,
even by inanimate objects, imposes itself upon our energy
field and our subtle perception.

We would also sense if other people were present, but it's
easier then to say that we heard breathing, or were aided

by our sense of smell. The fact remains that even our natural, moment-by-moment perception of our world is more complex than we might think. We're always employing something else, something extra, in our reading of what's around us, and this affects our action and interaction within the environment at any given time.

Part of what urges you to be a healer will probably be a natural, strong access to this something else. Training this extra factor in perception will lead you to sense, know, perceive, and perhaps (but only perhaps) hear and see other worlds as clearly and with the same organs of perception as those you employ in the outer, everyday world.

Knowing that energetic perception is aided by a factor in addition to the usual interaction of our five senses will help you to become subtly but accurately aware when you are healing, and to interpret this awareness to inform your healing sessions. The more open you stay to perception at the complex yet delicate subtle levels, the more you'll develop expertise in interpreting feeling and sensing. This sensing is precise and is often described as a "seeing" and "hearing" or even as a "touching," a "smelling," or a "tasting," although the physical senses are not directly involved.

Exercise
Sensing the Energy of Colors

Working with a friend or partner is always helpful when practicing healing development exercises of all kinds. It helps if you can prepare notes and help each other with the practicalities of the procedure, but it's also possible to work alone with a growth-of-sensitivity exercise such as this one. The ideal would be to first share it with an interested partner or friend and then to use it alone from time to time to train and sharpen your perceptions.

- Prepare some sheets of paper on which you have vividly painted or crayoned the colors of the rainbow. (Use one sheet per color. An 8½- by 11-inch or an 8½- by 11-inch sheet squared is about the right size.) It may not be easy to find an indigo paint or crayon, but try to have the basics of red, orange, yellow, green, blue, and violet. The violet should be a deep, rich color, not pale lavender or mauve.

- Preparing the sheets is part of the exercise. Take time and care with each one and, as you color them, allow yourself to feel the energy of the color. Maybe a certain color will have particular memories for you. Let these memories flow and sense the energy and atmosphere that goes with them, unless any are especially difficult or unhappy. (On the whole, if you have good, clear, positive colors, difficult memories will not be aroused by this exercise. But if this does happen leave that color aside until you have talked the memories through with a friend, partner, another healer, or a counselor. Transpersonal or psychosynthesis counselors would be particularly open to discussing issues that may arise from such an exercise as this. See Glossary, page 190.)

- Sense how each color affects you and where in your body you tend to respond to it. You may feel tension in muscles or organs, or you may experience mood changes that are linked to the stimuli of certain colors. Familiarize yourself with the energy that comes from the different colors and focus on the response and slight mood changes you feel in your own energy field.

- After a while, get your partner to arrange the colors in random order while you turn away or close your eyes. If you're working alone, shuffle the colors around on the floor or table while your eyes are closed.

- With your eyes still closed, get your partner to select one color at a time (or do so yourself) and hold it up to you, bringing it close to your outstretched hands and into your energy field around the level of either your solar plexus or your brow chakra until the colored sheet is about 6 inches away from you. See if you can sense the color on the paper without opening your eyes. Test whether you sense it better with your hands or when it's near your solar plexus or your brow chakra. You might find that you sense it first with your hands and also feel an answering response in either your solar plexus or your brow chakra or perhaps all of these.

- When you have done some initial work with sensing the colors one after the other, you may decide that you want to focus on a particular color in everyday life for a period of several days. One week you might choose violet, another orange, another green and so on, until you feel very familiar with the basic spectrum colors and their energies.

If this exercise works well for you with the clear, true colors of the spectrum, you can progress to more subtle shades, such as pinks, mauves, ambers, and different shades of green and blue, and experiment with the more neutral color range of brown, gray, mauve, black, and white.

Exercises
Meditations Using Color

Once you feel that you're becoming more sensitive to the energy of color in the outer world, it's a good idea to explore and use color in your inner world—seeing it in visual meditation with your inner eye, in your inner landscape. Here are two color visualizations or meditations that you can practice. The first also helps you to be more aware of the chakras and their areas of influence.

1. Meadow Meditation

- Making sure that you'll be undisturbed, sit or lie in a comfortable but symmetrically balanced position. Wrap yourself in a blanket for comfort and warmth if you wish, remembering that in meditation your body may lose heat. Unless you're sitting cross-legged or in a lotus position, don't cross your legs at the ankles or knees. Don't fold or cross your arms. Have the palms of your hands open and curved, and facing upwards. You can balance your hands, palms open and up, on your knees if you're sitting and on the floor beside you if you're lying down.

- Be aware of the rhythm of your breathing—don't force your breath or try to calm it. Simply allow it to find its own natural rhythm. Gradually bring that rhythm into your heart center or chakra, and sense how each in-breath and out-breath feeds, relaxes, and opens your heart chakra.

- Become aware of the column of subtle energy that runs through the center of your body. With your breath, follow this from just above the crown of your head down through the center of your body, out through your root chakra, and into the earth. Breathe with this direction of the energy flow for five or six breath sequences (in/out = one breath sequence), breathing in at the point just above your crown chakra and out into the earth, returning to the point above your crown chakra to take the next in-breath.

- Finish this part of the meditation on an exhalation into the earth. Then, visualizing a deep but soft, rosy red coming up from the earth on your next in-breath, breathe up as far as your root chakra and flood this chakra with the warming, energizing color, then breathe out again into the earth. As you breathe red up from the earth and into your root chakra for the third or fourth time, find yourself in a meadow in your inner landscape.

- The meadow is flooded with the wondrous shades of light and warmth that come from a rosy sunrise. The day is beginning and you're awake and alive to witness it. See the colors and the objects in your meadow, hear the sounds, smell the fragrances, touch the textures, and taste the tastes. Breathe naturally and normally. Rejoice in the gifts of earth and life as the rosy sunrise unfolds around you.

- From the meadow there is a clear path that leads along level ground and then beside a river with a bridge over it. Further on you can see that the path begins to climb, leading to hills and slopes beyond. As you follow the path to the bridge, the light around you becomes orangey, as the full morning sun prepares to break through.

- Breathing in this orange light, you come to the bridge over the river. As you stand on the bridge it seems that the whole world is bathed in orange. It reflects from the sky and from the water and bathes you. You can feel the power of the river beneath you. It is fast flowing and vital, and in the movement of the water every shade of orange and amber is visible, alive and at play. Trees grow on the riverbanks and for the moment they, too, seem to be orange. Even the birds in the branches and the rabbits at play on the riverbanks have an orangey glow about them, and the air is full of vigor and life force.

- From the bridge, the path begins to climb, sloping easily upward. Ahead of you, fascinatingly, you can see a place where the morning sun is shining directly on some randomly planted sunflowers. You follow the path to this spot, where you step aside for a few moments to savor the fragrance, color, and beauty of the sunflowers as they open themselves and stretch up to the sunlight. The morning yellow of the sun bathes you too, and for a few moments you live in a sunshiny yellow world, feeling yourself fed with the promise of midday warmth that the morning sun is already bringing.

- From this slightly raised point in your landscape you can see the path ahead and the path you've taken. No one else is about. There is only you, the light, the plants, animals, and the river. You feel fed with a sense of ownership and by the light of the sun that has become yellow, flooding over and into you. Digest all this for a few moments and then, as you decide to step back to the path and move on, let your hand brush over the face of a sunflower and notice how it becomes yellowed by the pollen dust, symbol of fecundity.

- The path goes on, climbing gently, and as it does you get more and more of an overview of your landscape. The vegetation around you is lush and green as you enter a wooded area. The sun shines through the leaves on the trees and, as you look up, the delicate, spring-like green of the light-filled leaves seems to become a part of you. You're in a green, leafy glade full of green light as the leaves filter the brightness of the sun on this beautiful day. Birds are singing and you feel your heart opening. You touch trees and plants and feel at one with them. The birdsong has a particularly melodious quality. As you bathe in the green light it seems that your heart sings too.

- Although the path has apparently only sloped easily and gently beneath your feet, as you come out of the wooded area you notice with surprise that you've come beyond the tree line onto rocky and slatey ground, with only intermittent sparse plants with shallow, parched roots. On this magical morning, however, the blue slate, bathed in sun, gives out a bright, clear color that glows like the blue of lapis lazuli.

- As you bathe in this color your throat chakra awakens, and as the world is your own, you sing and sound some clear notes, enjoying the echo that returns and reverberates around you. You can see over your landscape, back to the meadow where this path began, and on beyond the hills and slopes to the sea, which also glows blue and sparkles in the sunlight. The air is clear and the sounds you make are clear too. The blue light is cooling, cleansing, and invigorating at one and the same time.

- Now the path leads around to the more shady side of the slopes. Although you are at a vantage point in your landscape, the path is wide, safe, and undemanding. The shady side of the slopes, still with the blue slate covering them, has a glow of its own and you realize that you're being bathed in indigo light.

- You allow this color of mystery to feed into your being. As you do, you become particularly aware of the path you've walked today. You see where you've come from and then you see where the path leads—all the possibilities it has to offer and that you could choose to take. You feel an ethereal glow, a leap of spirit, a sense of joy and potential, a renewed perception of meaning in life.

- From this point the path leads on quite steeply. This last piece of your morning journey takes a little more exertion, but ahead of you there is a real vantage point where you know you'll feel lord or lady of all you survey. This point above you is bathed in a bright, deep violet light of its own. You long to bathe in it, and so the steepness of the path becomes easier.

- When you arrive at the high point there is a seat to rest on, right in the center of the violet light. As you sit there, you feel warmed by the sun but cleansed and invigorated by the violet light. You get a sense of communion with your higher self here and a renewed sense of purpose and meaning in your life. You feel energized and at peace.

- After a few minutes, you open your eyes to find that the intense violet light has faded and you're sitting in a sunny spot with a commanding view over your landscape and a clear stream trickling nearby. You refresh yourself with the clear water and know that you can either begin your journey back to the meadow where you began and descend to it gradually or that, if you just think yourself into the meadow, you'll be there instantly.

- Whichever way you choose, take yourself back to the meadow, and from there to an awareness of your breath in your heart center, and then to your body sitting or lying in your everyday surroundings. Let the petals of your heart chakra fold in, like those of a rose, gently but not tightly, protecting the center but allowing the fragrance of the rose to interact with the environment. Rest a while and then resume your normal, everyday activities.

2. Rainbow Meditation

- Making sure that you won't be undisturbed, sit or lie in a comfortable but symmetrically balanced position. Wrap yourself in a blanket for comfort and warmth if you wish, remembering that in meditation your body may lose heat. Unless you're sitting cross-legged or in a lotus position, don't cross your legs at the ankles or knees. Don't fold or cross your arms. Have the palms of your hands open and curved, and facing upward. You can balance your hands, palms open and up, on your knees if you're sitting and on the floor beside you if you're lying down.

- Be aware of the rhythm of your breathing—don't force your breath or try to calm it. Simply allow it to find its own natural rhythm. Gradually bring that rhythm into your heart center or chakra and sense how each in-breath and out-breath feeds, relaxes, and opens your heart chakra.

- Become aware of the column of subtle energy that runs through the center of your body. With your breath, follow this from just above the crown of your head down through the center of your body, out through your root chakra, and into the earth. Breathe with this direction of the energy flow for five or six breath sequences (in/out = one breath sequence), breathing in at the point just above your crown chakra and out into the earth, returning to the point above your crown chakra to take the next in-breath.

- Finish this part of the meditation on an exhalation into the earth. As you breathe up again, focus on your heart chakra before finding yourself in a meadow in your inner landscape. Take the opportunity to activate your inner senses, see the colors and the objects around you, hear the sounds, smell the fragrances, touch the textures, and taste the tastes. Breathe naturally and normally. From your meadow you can see your inner landscape opening out and, as you look, you see that there's a rainbow, bright, translucent, and sparkling. You also see that there's a point not too far away where it seems that you can, in this inner world of yours, enter the place where the rainbow colors join the earth.

- Go to this place and find that you can indeed stand at the center of the rainbow, bathed in all its colors. Feel the quality of translucent light drenched with color. Accept the rainbow colors into your own body, feel them healing you, and sense your response to them. The whole spectrum is here: red, orange, yellow, green, blue, indigo, and violet.

- When you've had enough of this magical, energizing and healing experience, step out of the rainbow, return to the place where you entered your meadow, and from here to an awareness of your body and the rhythm of your breath in your heart chakra. Let the petals of your heart chakra close in gently, protecting your heart energy without tightly sealing this center. When you feel grounded and centered again, return to your normal, everyday activities.

Exercise
Mentally Sending and Receiving Colors

This exercise works best with a partner or maybe a small group of interested people. If this is totally impossible, some suggestions for using it by yourself are also given.

- Sit opposite your partner, or facing a small group. Each of you should begin by becoming aware of your breathing, letting the rhythm find its own level and then using the breath at your heart chakra level to activate your heart energy. This creates the atmosphere in which to work.
- One person then tries to visualize one of six of the spectrum colors clearly and strongly, projecting the visualization out into the room or toward the partner or group. The colors are: red, orange, yellow, green, blue, and violet.
- The partner or group try to sense the energy of the color and where in the body it is received or what area of the body it activates. Receiving the energy and feeling it in the body is initially more important than being accurate about which color is being transmitted, but if you practice together, an accuracy in sensing the color itself will gradually grow.
- Although people vary in where they might be activated in the body by a certain color, it's most usual to receive red in the root or heart chakra areas, orange at sacral or throat, yellow at solar plexus, brow, or crown, green at heart or root, blue at throat or sacral, and violet at crown, brow, or solar plexus. The chakras may feel

activated or organs in the area of the chakras may
respond to the colors. Energization may be felt at the
front and/or the back of the body.

- If you have a small group working together, a variation
on this exercise is to have one person sitting in the
center of the group with the whole group visualizing the
color. Your color sheets are useful here: the group waits
until the central person has their eyes shut; then a color
sheet can be held up to the group as a silent signal about
which color to focus on. After three or four minutes,
senders and receivers can comment on the atmosphere
and reactions produced by the focus on each particular
color.

- If you can only work alone, you can use the technique of
invocation to activate this exercise for yourself. Although
you'll know what color you're invoking, you can still
sense its energies and qualities, receive it in your body
and perceive the atmosphere it brings into your
environment.

- Work with one color at a time, maybe one each day or
every other day. Read the section on invocation on page
48. Decide which color you want to work with, do the
heart center breathing recommended above, close your
eyes, and say something simple such as, "I invoke the
color orange in a pure, healing, and energizing form,"
and then spend a few moments bathing in the color and
noting your reactions to it.

Exercise
Color Healing Sequence

This healing sequence is an expansion of the earlier healing
sequences (see pages 35 and 38), adding color to what has
gone before. Practice first with a partner if possible.

- Choose whether you want to work with your patient sitting (see page 35) or lying down (see page 38). Carefully reread the instructions for the healing sequence you've chosen. Pay particular attention to your preparation with running energy and making a healing invocation.

- Information about the alter major chakra is given on page 94 and you may like to include this in your healing sequence now. Remember that it has its positive electrical energy point at the back of the head and its negative one at the front in the region of the nose. Therefore at this chakra you need to remember to put your left hand at the front and your right hand at the back. It's usually best if you go to the alter major after you've dealt with the crown. Then if you want to stand on the other side of your patient, it's easy to do so without needing to change position more than once.

- As you go through the chakra points and heal the areas of the body requiring special attention, interpret the energies you pick up from your patient as color. Think of each color as you're working and gradually have the courage to visualize color flowing through your hands into the chakras.

  As you gain experience and sensitivity, you'll instinctively know which auric colors need balancing or feeding, and whether a particular color is almost nonexistent. But to begin with, you cannot go wrong if, as you heal each chakra point, you visualize the principal color for that chakra clearly and translucently, seeing it as stained glass appears when sunlight passes through it. (The colors are rosy red for the root, orange for the sacral, yellow for the solar plexus, green for the heart, blue for the throat, indigo for the brow, violet for the crown, and a rich, clear, translucent, reddish brown for the alter major, if you have decided to include it.)

- For bodily areas requiring special attention, soft reds are warming, pink is comforting, orange and amber are energizing, yellow awakens and lightens, green soothes and encourages flow where there may be blockage, blue cools and quiets pain, and indigo and violet aid relaxation and calm any fear or panic.

- When you've finished the healing session, carry out the energetic separation and rounding off as for all healing sequences.

As you practice this exercise and other healing sequences, you'll begin to realize that sometimes your hands are picking up information from your patient's energy field and chakras, and sometimes they're aiding the healing flow to come through you to the patient. There's quite a difference in energy between sensing your patients' energy fields and actually channeling healing. When you feel sensations in the palms of your hands like prickling, heat, or coolness, you're usually reading what's going on in your patient's energy field or aura. When you feel a flow through your hands and fingers or are drawn intuitively to certain body areas, this is the healing flow using you as its channel and for its direction.

As you go on to use more and more specific healing procedures, it's important to endeavor to make this differentiation, so that you can be more involved in reading or sensing what's required and deciding which healing exercises to use to augment the healing session.

Chakras and colors are important in our energy fields. Learning to sense color helps to develop your subtle perceptions as a healer. The energy field is also made up of layers, related to and interacting with the chakras, and each also having its own color and electrical energy. These layers are often referred to as subtle bodies. The next chapter describes them and their functions.

Chapter 6

The Auric Layers

Robert's story—Subtle energy system—The etheric body—
The astral body—The feeling body—The mental body—
The higher mental body—The soul, ketheric, or causal body—
Wholeness of being—Exercises

ROBERT'S STORY

Robert was a keen amateur tennis player. He was attracted to learning about healing ever since a friend with healing gifts treated a strained leg tendon for him. It healed quickly and strongly, in time for Robert to take part in a tournament to which he'd been particularly looking forward. He felt there was no real reason why he should assume that he too might be able to heal as a result of his experience, but the idea persisted. He decided to come to some of my healing practice sessions for developing healers.

When Robert received healing from others in the group, he felt very moved and was aware of something happening within and around him. When he gave healing to others, they felt a strong sense of healing surrounding them.

Despite these reports and encouragement, and although he never missed a group session and assiduously practiced everything I could teach, for a long time Robert said that he experienced nothing at all when he was endeavoring to be a healing channel. He had to rely on the encouraging reports from others.

When Robert was introduced to the first stage of sensing the subtle energy field (see page 14) at his first session with the group, he was fascinated and excited. When healing, he could always sense the edge of his patient's energy field, but he wanted more and felt disappointed with his own perceptions of his development.

When we worked with training color perception, Robert began to sense the different color vibrations and energies, and felt more secure about accurately locating each chakra. He insisted that much of this was common sense or very transient. Obviously, deprecating his own gifts and anything he might briefly sense did not help him in his desire to develop and train his subtle sensitivities. To want or expect too much too soon can be an obstacle to laying the basic foundation on which to build.

While working with and discussing subtle anatomy and the broader subtle energies of the aura, things ultimately began to fall into place for Robert. He felt perfectly at home with the idea of different layers and planes, and related strongly to the notion of sensing subtle textures. As a veil lifted for him, he was at last able to value the very multi-faceted nature of perception. I felt that Robert had finally opened that layer of his heart chakra that enables entry to the contemplative state in which all subtle perceptions are at their strongest. When this happens—and it's worth persevering until it does—subtle experience becomes more vivid and meaningful and expands effortlessly. (The exercise on page 124 supports and assists this process.)

I've included Robert's story here because he's typical of many for whom the opening of subtle perception happens very gradually, with many doubts along the way. Although the ultimate aim must always be to return to simplicity, the more areas you learn about and explore, even very tentatively, the more opportunities there are for your perception of subtle energies to develop and for you to find the key that enables a growth of confidence.

SUBTLE ENERGY SYSTEM

As I've already outlined (see page 87), the chakras are wheels and centers of light, color, and energy. They interpenetrate with the physical body, and affect and are affected by our physical, mental, emotional, and spiritual states. They carry links to the body's glandular system and are, in a sense, refined glands.

There are myriad subtle energy pathways interpenetrating with our physical bodies. They're called meridians and nadis (see also page 28) and are like refined arteries and veins. The nadis run everywhere, like numberless branching and intersecting minor roads or pathways over a territory. The meridians are more major pathways finely connecting the major organs to each other and carrying energy from the major organs throughout the whole of our complex physical and interconnecting subtle systems.

The eight major chakras occur where there is major production or crossing of nadis and meridians. Numerous other minor chakras form where there is a less busy production and fewer crossing points. Most of these minor chakras are connected to organs of the body, such as the spleen, the liver, kidneys, and pancreas.

The eyes, ears, hands, feet, and bony structure of the head carry links to all the major and minor chakras in the body. They are used as focus points for imparting finely tuned healing in disciplines such as iridology, metamorphic technique, reflexology, and cranial osteopathy.

THE ETHERIC BODY

In esoteric teaching, there are seven layers to our total being and energy field, including the physical body. Each organ of the body has a subtle counterpart, and the sum total of meridians, nadis, chakras, and subtle organ counterparts forms the "body" or auric layer closest to the physical. This is known as the etheric body or layer. (Names for the differ-

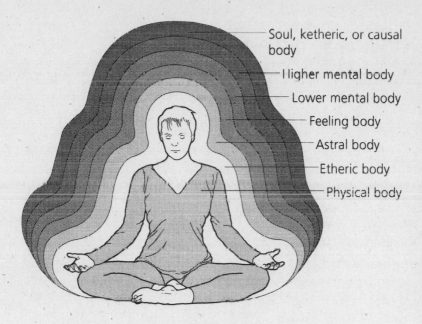

The physical body and the six layers of the auric field.

ent layers, bodies, or planes vary throughout esoteric teaching. Here I use the terms that I've been taught.) It's a subtle double of the physical layer and the densest of the subtle bodies. In disease, the etheric body has to repair itself before the physical organs can return to normal. Most healing for the physical body is received first at the etheric level. When this is balanced and invigorated, the healing permeates the physical level body.

When any part of the physical body is amputated or removed, its etheric essence remains. The phantom limb is a medically accepted fact. The etheric body may be very traumatized and need intensive healing but it remains whole. Losing a physical organ does not mean losing its etheric counterpart. This is one of the reasons why the physical body is able to adapt and carry on functioning even when a relatively important organ has been removed.

With the modern drugs of allopathic medicine, we live under a delusion that healing can happen quite quickly. Certainly many unpleasant symptoms can be eased, but when symptoms disappear the journey of healing is not necessarily complete, especially for the etheric body. Recovery from illness needs time, rest, and tender loving care, whether the presenting symptoms have been miraculously cured or suppressed or not.

There's no denying that allopathy has produced many breakthroughs in healing, but the subtle bodies have their own healing rhythm and may be adversely affected by the strong medications that remove physical symptoms. Resting when ill is sometimes seen as weak or undignified, but our present way of life can be too demanding for our intricate constitutions, and society often requires that we push ourselves too far. As healers bent on understanding the whole spectrum of healing, we need to help our patients honor the healing process by taking the time to heal that's required by the etheric body.

When the etheric body is sensed, it feels tingly, prickly, and "electric." Its color is orangey. This layer has strong links to the sacral chakra and the lymphatic glands. The plane of being to which the etheric body helps us connect is known as the etheric plane. It's full of echoes of the experiences we have on the physical plane. When working as a healer or to develop spiritual perception, it can be important to be aware of keeping the etheric body, and the immediately surrounding etheric plane, bright and active. It can

become rather heavy and, instead of being a bright, energized web around us, become more like a dust-filled cobweb.
The exercise on page 130 describes how to keep personal
links to the etheric body and plane working at their optimum
level for you.

THE ASTRAL BODY

Moving out from the physical body, the second subtle layer
or body, known as the astral body, consists of subtle flowing
energies. Its color is yellow gold, rose, or a clear, slightly
electric, silvery blue. It has strong links to the solar plexus
chakra and the adrenal glands. When sensed, it feels cool
and fluid. The plane of being to which it helps us connect is
known as the astral plane.

A frequently reported aspect of near-death experience is
of being in another part of the room, usually high up near
the ceiling, watching what's happening to the physical
body. Those who have survived serious accidents have
reported watching their physical body being rescued or
treated, while their consciousness or essence waits at a
distance, away from the physical pain and distress. In these
experiences the awareness is withdrawn to the astral body
or plane.

Many people become attracted to the spiritual path
because of the possibility of learning astral travel. In this
altered state of consciousness, journeys through time and
space, and even bilocation, become possible. Anyone who
wants to work specifically with esoteric development of the
astral body should consult a well-established esoteric school
or find a trusted teacher.

The higher astral plane, as described by esotericists and
sensitives, is very beautiful. It has flowing landscapes and
healing temples. It is the plane where there is a loving
contact with guides, helpers, and angelic beings and the one

where we are met and welcomed when, in death, we finally leave our physical bodies.

Lower layers of the astral plane are less attractive. Thought forms and negative entities populate these regions. Some of the experiences of bad drug trips and schizophrenia can come from a vulnerability that precipitates an unwanted breakthrough into these realms. These vulnerable states usually mean that the chakra stems have become too open, with the natural flow from petals to stem being upset.

The chakra stems open intermittently to eliminate subtle toxins, but when they become too open they may not seal themselves properly or control this natural flow. An open stem can attract an unwanted infiltration of energies from the lower astral plane and result in mental confusion, frightening and vivid visions, and irrational promptings. Damaged stems need subtle healing energy, as from a healer, to help them repair. Some healers and psychic workers choose to specialize in working with people who have become disoriented by these influences.

THE FEELING BODY

The third subtle layer, moving outward from the physical body, is the feeling body. It has strong links to the heart chakra and the thymus gland (linked to growth and maturation). The feeling body is a very pale, light green in color. When sensed, it feels warmer, softer, and less fluid than the astral body but is also very full of vitality.

When awareness is projected into the feeling body, perceptions are considerably sharpened and heightened. People and objects may be experienced in a special way. Tapping into the feeling body layer enables us to enter a state known as contemplation, which is a deep level of meditation (see page 124). In this state there is full identification with other people, trees, rocks, plants, crystals, or animals.

We experience from within and sense the nature of other beings and life forms, sharing, as much as it is ever possible to share, the nature of other humans or life forms and their rhythms and life cycles.

It's the feeling body that enables the ultimate, mystical experience of total oneness or unity with the universe, described by contemplatives, mystics, and poets. Those earth-shattering, totally satisfying moments of unity with a lover where you lose yourselves in each other are also one of the products of connection with the feeling body.

Using more heart colors in your decor, clothing, or environment helps to awaken and open access to your feeling body. Robert's (see page 114) breakthrough in subtle sensing and perception came when dogged persistence with his healing development strengthened his link to his feeling body.

THE MENTAL BODY

The fourth level out from the physical body is the mental body. When sensed, it has a fluid but tingly texture. It is reflective, and glows with very subtle shades of blue, silver, and turquoise. These are the colors of the throat chakra, to which it has a strong link. The glandular connection is to the thyroid.

As its name implies, the mental body is partly connected to intellect and abstract thought, to the world of ideas, conceptual blueprints, and archetypes. It links us to those unseen patterns, subtle nuances, and barely heard sounds that are aspects of complex communication. It enables us to apprehend, name, and implement certain volatile and abstract aspects of the universe, and make use of them in life and incarnation. This includes our integral awareness of, and struggle with, divine principles or qualities. We feel a true sense of human potential when our societies reflect qualities such as peace, love, justice, respect, and the right relationship to power. We struggle to define these in life. Being in touch with our mental bodies and the mental plane helps us find integrity.

Healing for the throat chakra and mental body helps concepts to change. If a patient is frightened or convinced that an illness, condition, or lifestyle resulting from chronic disease or impairment cannot be improved in any way, a new, more positive attitude can emerge, enabling greater symbolic understanding.

THE HIGHER MENTAL BODY

This is the fifth layer working outward from the physical body. It's linked to the brow chakra and to the pineal gland. The higher mental body is of a supremely light and subtle substance. It reflects deep indigo and amethyst colors and when sensed is filmy, sheer, ethereal, pulsating, and cool.

The higher mental body is the "garment" we wear for our highest levels of meditational experience, communication with other planes, and intense moments of inspiration.

The mental plane is filled with sheer and pulsating waves. The inspiration that gives birth to ideas originates here, before it becomes clothed with language or form. It is the plane of divine principle, pure archetypal impulses and of the archangelic beings: Michael, Uriel, Raphael, and Gabriel. (See Glossary, page 189, for more detail on pure archetypal impulses and angels.)

THE SOUL, KETHERIC, OR CAUSAL BODY

These are alternative names for the sixth and final subtle body, encountered when moving outward through the auric field from the physical. It's linked to the crown chakra and the pituitary gland. It glows with intense but pale and fine violet light. When sensed, it feels flowing and silky. It has a warm, soft glow.

The ketheric body is an evolutionary imprint or reflection from the soul. In incarnation, this layer can affect us through those subtle memories from other lives that cause us to react to positive or negative stimuli in a manner not directly explicable in terms of our present life experience. Unexpectedly intense or so-called irrational fears, free floating anxieties, *déjà vu* experiences, and exceptional giftedness are all examples of the interpenetration of the soul, ketheric, or causal body.

This layer of the auric field holds the imprint of the learning intentions we have made for this lifetime. Connection with this body and plane will help us to see a higher pattern, purpose, and direction in our lives.

WHOLENESS OF BEING

Working with the wider energy field surrounding each one of us begins (as in "Sensing the Energy Field," page 14) with an overall electrical sensing. It progresses through an awareness of chakras as energy and color points, interpenetrating with our physical bodies, to an ever clearer impression of the distinct layers within our aura of being.

The more we feel into and accept the multifaceted and rainbow nature of our wider substance, the more we realize the many complexities that can affect our health and well-being. We are finely balanced. Channeled healing energy is equally finely attuned and infiltrates all our layers, energy points, subtle bodies, and layers. Maximizing our potential makes our response to life and incarnation total and healthful. Glimpsing the wonder of our wider fineness of being also helps us, as healers, to appreciate the refined nature of our extended potential for perception.

Channeled healing automatically seeks out and balances the different subtle levels, but as your healing expertise develops, you may want to carry out more conscious and specific healing techniques. Giving extra attention to the etheric body, for instance, strengthens the potential for healing to manifest at the physical level and for depleted organs to be energized. Specific healing for the astral body may help people who grieve, fear death, are mentally ill, or suffer with bad dreams or nightmares.

Consciously treating the feeling body will help people who want to be more perceptive and open to wider aspects of being. It will also help those who are too open to unseen influences and who tend to take the weight of the world on their shoulders.

Healing the mental body will help people who fear to speak their own truth or who are out of touch with the real value of their own integrity. For those who live in too abstract a world, it will help with the ability to know what they are feeling, while they're feeling it.

Working with the higher mental body will help people connect with the energy of the true spirit of their being and to find wider meaning in life. Healing for the soul, ketheric, or causal body helps those who feel directionless to find life's purpose once more and to feel connected to something higher but personal. It can help those who are going through personal tragedy to feel less abandoned and to find a perspective for what has happened.

Exercise
Enabling the Contemplative Level of Perception

This exercise is good for helping the development of a healer's sensitivity and ability to "read" the patient.

You need a plant, a crystal, and connection with a tree, an animal, or another person. It takes practice to establish this

level of the heart chakra as one that will open for you whenever you want to attune to different levels of awareness and
perception. You are recommended to repeat the exercise at
least once a week but not more than every other day over a
period of time. Whichever option you've chosen from plant,
crystal, tree, animal, or other person, work with that first
choice two or three times, so that you can get a sense of
progression. It's important to vary your experience by moving on to another available option and staying with that for
two or three times. Keep up a variety, but after trying new
options, always return to former ones.

Before you begin the process below, make your selection.
If you're going to use a plant or crystal, have it near you. If
you're choosing to attune to a small domestic animal, you
can take it on your knee or simply make sure it's in the same
room. If you're attuning to another person, sit opposite
them, if possible, attuning to each other at the same time. If
you're attuning to an outdoor animal or a tree, you'll need
to be able to sit or, perhaps in summer, lie down in its vicin-
ity. Always try to touch the animal or tree before you begin
this attunement.

During the exercise, the plant, crystal, animal, tree, or
person you've chosen to work with is referred to as an ally.
The practice leads you to a point where you endeavor to let
your energy field blend with the ally and let the energy field
of the ally flow into you. It's important to make sure that
your chosen ally is one you feel comfortable with.

The flowing of one energy into the other is a state of
contemplation. It's important as you first practice this exer
cise to allow the contemplative state to last for only two or
three minutes. If you know that there's a time limit at this
stage, part of you will honor it and you'll move back into a
lighter state of meditation after the allowed time, without the
need to use a timer. If you feel uncertain of this, you can
prerecord the instructions for this practice, leaving a two- or
three-minute gap on your tape before you speak the next

words. As you grow used to the sensation, you can expand the time up to ten or fifteen minutes.

Remember that contemplation is a deep meditative state. Allow plenty of time for the transition from contemplation through ordinary level meditation to everyday life.

- Making sure that you'll be undisturbed, sit or lie comfortably with your body in a symmetrical position and your back well supported, if necessary. Sit in a cross-legged or lotus posture (see page 183), if you wish, but otherwise don't cross your legs at your ankles or knees. Have your arms and hands by your side with your palms curved open and facing upward, if lying down, or hands balanced on your knees, palms curved open and facing upward, if sitting. Pay particular attention to the balance and alignment of your head and neck, since this helps energy circulate freely through your chakras.
- Close your eyes and become aware of the rhythm of your breathing. After a few moments, change to breathing for grounding and energy running (see page 16).
- When you feel what should by now be the familiar sense of becoming calm and grounded, focus your breathing into your heart chakra. Sense your heart chakra like a rose that's about to open. Its outer petals are spring green, while there's a promise of a tender rosy pink within and, at the very center, a touch of gold. It has a delicate fragrance. The colors are translucent and ethereal, yet the rose itself has substance. With each in-breath and out-breath the petals unfold, releasing more and more fragrance, and the heart center colors surround you. As the center of the rose reveals itself, you see that the base of each petal has a delicate amethyst light and tinge, and then a depth of gold in the center that's almost like a gateway inviting you to go deeper and further. Your heart center is pulsating and turning.

- Let yourself gradually be drawn into the golden center of your heart chakra. Sense a fine, golden light spreading around you and within you, illuminating your body and your being. Sense an expansion of your awareness. Let this sense of expansion move out toward the plant, crystal, person, animal, or tree that you've chosen to work with on this occasion.

- Let the fine golden light surround your contemplative ally (plant, crystal, person, animal, or tree). Breathe it out toward them, let it surround them and then breathe it back into your heart chakra. Feel your rhythm joining with theirs, sense the life force of your ally, be at one with it—have a sense of unity and sharing with it. Let yourself know, in your heart, what it is to be that ally until you are a part of it and it's a part of you. Sustain this part of the meditation for only two or three minutes at first.

- Gradually draw the fine golden light back toward yourself. Feel it containing and surrounding you. Become aware again of the rose fragrance and the delicate greens and pinks of the petals of the rose of your heart. Feel a pulsing rhythm within your heart center that links with the central rhythm of the universe . . . with rhythms of earth and sea . . . with currents of air . . . and with the flicker of flames in a gentle warming fire. Feel your body being healed and vitalized.

- Gradually let the petals of your heart chakra begin to fold in again. Let them just relax, so that the petals retain a resilience, without being too tightly closed or too widely open and vulnerable. See spring green light all around and over the flower of your heart chakra.

- Then, through the rhythm of your breath, return to an awareness of your body, your contact with the ground, and your normal everyday surroundings. Visualize a cross of white light in a circle of white light over your heart chakra and draw a cloak of white light with a hood right around you. Feel your feet firmly in contact with the ground and refocus into the outer world thoroughly before resuming your normal tasks.

Exercise
Enhancing Your Subtle Body Layers

This exercise helps to cleanse, strengthen, and differentiate your subtle bodies. It is energizing, healing, and protective, but will also help as you train your perception to sense, and perhaps eventually see, the six subtle layers of the aura that extend beyond the physical body.

Seven bands of light and color are breathed around your body from left to right, starting and ending at your feet, then seven more from the back of your body to the front, also starting and ending at your feet. The colors are deep rose pink, amber, golden yellow, spring green, lapis lazuli blue, indigo, and deep violet, and should be visualized or imagined as vibrant and translucent—like stained glass when sunlight passes through it.

Red links to the root chakra and energizes the physical body, orange to the sacral and energizes the etheric body, yellow to the solar plexus and energizes the astral body, green to the heart and energizes the feeling body, blue to the throat and energizes the lower mental body, indigo to the brow and energizes the higher mental body, and violet to the crown and energizes the ketheric, causal, or soul body.

Eventually you can do this meditation in almost any position or situation, but first practice it standing, if possible, or sitting on an upright chair.

- Stand easily and comfortably. Pay attention to the balance of your head on your neck. Place your feet comfortably apart; don't tense your shoulders or lock your knees. Relax any tension in the lower part of your body and rock your pelvis a little until you have a relaxed stance.

- Before beginning to visualize the colors, pay attention to your breathing. Imagine a breath that starts underneath your feet on the in-breath and travels up your left side, close to your body, to the crown of your head. Here you start the out-breath, which goes down the right side of your body to the starting position under your feet. Practice these breaths until the rhythm is flowing easily.
- Now, begin the light and color breaths. Visualizing deep rose pink light, breathe a band of this color up your left side on the in-breath, keeping the color band close to your physical body. At the crown of your head, change to the out-breath and take the deep rose color down the right side of your body, letting it join under your feet.
- Do the same with each color in turn, moving slightly further out from your body as you breathe each new band until you're surrounded with a rainbow of colored light. Light and color can interpenetrate with physical matter, so visualize the bands of light lying as evenly under your feet as around the rest of your body. Once you've established the spectrum of light around you in this direction, continue to breathe evenly.
- The next step is to breathe the light and color bands around you from back to front. Again, you start under your feet, with deep rose pink. Breathe it up the back of your body to the crown of your head on the in-breath and down the front of your body to join under your feet on the out-breath. End with violet, as before.
- When you have breathed all the bands of light and color from side to side and back to front, continue to breathe evenly and let each band of color expand and join around you until it forms an egg shape. Imagine a Russian doll effect. You are in the center, surrounded by seven eggs of light and color. Feel strengthened, energized, protected, and secure.

- Before you take up your normal tasks once more, visualize a silver egg of light enclosing the other seven. In this way, you take light and energy with you wherever you go, but are less vulnerable to any unwanted impingement from the outer world.

When you know this exercise well, it's not always necessary to go through the complete breathing and visualization— though it's a good meditative practice in itself. At any time when you feel vulnerable or in need of an energy boost, you can merely visualize the seven eggs of light and color surrounding you, with the final egg of silver as a container for the energy and a way of absorbing all the healing effect light and color can bring. This is also a good exercise to teach to your patients.

Exercise
Cleansing Your Etheric Field

Since healers are often vulnerable to picking things up from the environment or even from the psyches of their patients, this is an important practice for the maintenance of healer health. It's similar to the aura combing stage of the basic healing sequence (see page 37), but this version is done through visualization and is an exercise for maintaining personal vitality and clarity. It keeps the etheric web fresh and vital.

You can do the exercise lying down (good times are just before you sleep or on waking), sitting, or standing. One of my trainee healers said she used it frequently in a bus line or on a train platform!

- Become aware of your breathing and your body. Become aware of the energy field that stretches beyond your body, especially the first or etheric layer, that's near to your physical body and emanates out from it.

- Imagine that you have a small brush, perhaps similar to a toothbrush, dipped in light, and that you're gently but systematically brushing this first layer of your subtle bodies with light. Imagine it as a fine web that fills with light as you brush. Imagine your body gently enclosed in and protected by this light-filled mesh and that anything that might have been sticky or heavy around you has now been cleansed away.
- Let your heart chakra petals gently close in and then either go to sleep, if you're doing this as the last thing at night, or begin your day with new energy for whatever is coming next in your life.

Exercise
Sensing the Auric Layers

For this exercise you really need a partner to work with—although you can endeavor to use your hands to sense your own subtle bodies. Remember that the intense layers of the auric field are usually all held within 4 to 6 inches of the physical body, so each movement outward into the six bodies beyond the physical is very slight. It is an attunement to the next level of being.

Though the subtle bodies may be explained, and clairvoyantly seen, as being layer upon layer, to some extent they interpenetrate or intermix with each other. Sensing them is not so much about discovering where one layer ends and another begins as about developing an awareness of the energies that coexist around us.

- Let your partner sit in a chair or lie down, face upward, on couch or floor. Begin by grounding and running energy (see page 16). Approach your partner from the front, back, or either side if they're sitting, and from the side and above if lying. Rub the palms of your hands

together to awaken your hand chakras. Ask permission
to gently place your hands on your partner's physical
body. Make sure they're resting very lightly and then
visit several positions on the body, say the shoulders,
solar plexus, knees, and the calves or feet. Be aware of
the warmth and energy of the physical body, which gives
out a faint, deep, rosy red color.

- When you can feel this warmth and perhaps sense or
  even glimpse the soft redness, move your hands very
  slightly out from your partner's body so that you're still
  very close to the body but not touching it. Try to pick up
  a prickly sensation with an impression of a clear but
  delicate orange or amber color. The prickly, electrically
  tingling layer is the etheric layer.

- If you have difficulty sensing the etheric layer generally,
  hold your hands at either side of your partner's body at
  the same level as the sacral chakra, and only move
  elsewhere when you've picked up the electrical, tingling
  sensation. (While sensing the subtle body layers you can
  move back and rub your hands together again, or you
  can just gradually let your hands move outward very
  slightly, as you endeavor to sense each stratum.)

- Move a little way out again and run your hands over,
  but off, the body. You're now seeking to experience or
  sense the astral layer. Remember that this layer is
  smooth, flowing, and cool. Sense the change in texture.
  The color can vary from a pale, golden yellow through
  rose pink to a silvery blue. If, initially, you have difficulty
  in picking this body up, hold your hands at either side of
  your partner's body at the solar plexus level, where the
  vibrations of the astral body tend to be strongest.

- Once more, move your hands out very slightly. You're
  now moving into the feeling body, the third layer out
  from the physical body. This layer is vital but less fluid
  than the astral body. It has a softer, warmer texture and

glows with delicate light green colors. It can be sensed most strongly on a level with the heart chakra, to which it's strongly connected.

- The fourth layer, moving outward from the physical body, is the mental body. With connections to the throat chakra, it is sensed most strongly at and around throat chakra level. The mental body is fluid and tingly in texture. It reflects fine blue, silver, and turquoise colors.

- The fifth layer or level of the subtle bodies, connected to the brow chakra and therefore most strongly sensed around that area, is the higher mental body. This has a supremely light and subtle texture, and glows with pale indigo and amethyst. Its texture is filmy, sheer, pulsating, and cool.

- The sixth and final level of the subtle bodies is the variously titled soul, ketheric, or causal body. It's linked to the crown chakra and may be best sensed around that area of the body. It radiates a pale but intense violet light and its texture is flowing and silky, with a soft warm glow.

- When you've finished working with your partner, make an energetic separation (see page 19). It's essential to do this, even if you're about to exchange your positions.

When you first try this exercise, you may feel some sensations clearly and others only vaguely or not at all. At first you may feel nothing except the warm radiance from the physical body of your partner. Keep practicing! Don't give up! These subtle perceptions have a habit of suddenly becoming clear, easy, and natural but can only do so if you persist with the exercises.

Exercises
Drawing Out Negative Energy

This is a useful healing exercise as a variation on those that principally use the chakra points or work more directly with points of pain, discomfort, or disease. Called chelation, it helps to blend, balance, integrate, and improve the flow of all the fine layers and points in the subtle anatomy of the being. Chelation means *drawing out.* It draws out toxins and gently sorts out any tangles or knots in the totality of our being. In practice, it's simple to use, while its effects are deep and wide throughout the physical and subtle energy system.

As we've already seen, the chakra points reflect imbalances in the total being and are receptive points for healing of all kinds. But there are other points on the body where any weakness, distortion, or confusion in the flow of the subtle energies will show up, and where receptivity to healing and adjustment is strong. Among these are the points used for chelation, which are beneath the feet, in the knees and the knee joint, where the legs join the body, in the hips, at the waist, at the wrists, at the elbows, at the shoulders, at the neck, and at the crown of the head.

Chelation is most easily channeled when your patient or a partner with whom you're working is lying down, but may also be given when the patient is sitting on a chair. In chelation, as in other healing sequences, remember to lay your hands very lightly on your patient. Touching too heavily or firmly or leaning on the body will not enhance your patient's healing experience!

Chelation can be practiced by one healer, or by two working in partnership. Always prepare for giving a chelation as you would for any other healing, but note the additional preparation and attunement needed if you're working with another healer to channel healing together to one patient.

1. One Healer, Patient Lying Down

- Settle your patient on the floor, couch, or bed. If possible, you should be able to move completely around your patient and be able to stand at the head and at the feet. Make your initial healing preparation and attunement of grounding and running energy and invocation (see pages 16 and 48).
- Begin by standing behind your patient's head and then, having asked for permission to touch the body lightly, gently place both hands on your patient's crown. Hold your hands still until you sense a quietness or balancing happening—or for two or three minutes.
- Now, keeping your right hand in touch with the crown of the head, move your left hand down to the base of your patient's neck at the left-hand side, where it joins the body. Endeavor to sense the energy flow and balance happening between your hand points.
- When a balance or change seems to have happened, or after about two minutes, move your right hand down to join your left at the base of the left-hand side of your patient's neck. Move your feet so that you're not stretching to reach. Basically, during a chelation, you'll walk right around your patient, from left to right. A moment or so after moving your right hand down to join your left at the base of the neck, shift your left hand out to your patient's left shoulder and again sense how the flow between your hands helps to balance, move, and change the energy.

This sequence of movement, where you heal the flow between two points and then let your hands join on the same point before separating them again, is essential to a successful chelation.

- After about two minutes, or when you sense a positive healing change, move your right hand to join your left at the shoulder. When they've been very briefly at the same point together, move your left hand down to your client's left elbow. Wait again, either for two minutes or until you sense change, and bring your right hand to join your left at the left elbow of your patient. Move your left hand to your patient's left wrist and continue as before.

With the healing pauses, the sequence continues:

- Your right hand joins your left at your patient's left wrist and your left hand moves to your patient's waist.
- After two minutes of healing flow, your right hand joins your left at your patient's left waist and then your left hand moves down to your patient's lower hip.
- After two minutes of healing flow, your right hand joins your left at your patient's left lower hip and then your left hand moves down to your patient's left knee.
- After two minutes of healing flow, your right hand joins your left at your patient's left knee and then your left hand moves down to your patient's left ankle.
- After two minutes of healing flow, your right hand joins your left at your patient's left ankle and your left hand moves down to the sole of your patient's left foot.
- After two minutes of healing flow, your right hand joins your left on the sole of your patient's foot and your left hand moves to the sole of your patient's right foot.
- After two minutes of healing flow, your right hand joins your left on the sole of your patient's right foot and your left hand moves to your patient's right ankle.
- After two minutes of healing flow, your right hand joins your left at your patient's right ankle and your left hand moves to your patient's right knee.
- After two minutes of healing flow, your right hand

moves to join your left at your patient's right knee and your left hand moves to your patient's lower, right hip.

- After two minutes of healing flow, your right hand moves to join your left at your patient's right hip and your left hand moves to your patient's right waist.
- After two minutes of healing flow, your right hand moves to join your left at your patient's right waist and your left hand moves to your patient's right wrist.
- After two minutes of healing flow, your right hand moves to join your left at your patient's right wrist and your left hand moves to your patient's right elbow.
- After two minutes of healing flow, your right hand joins your left at your patient's right elbow and your left hand moves to your patient's right shoulder.
- After two minutes of healing flow, your right hand moves to join your left at your patient's right shoulder and your left hand moves to the base of your patient's neck on the right-hand side of the body.
- After two minutes of healing flow, your right hand joins your left at your patient's right-hand side base of neck and your left hand moves to the crown of your patient's head.
- After two minutes of healing flow, your right hand moves to join your left at the crown of your patient's head. You have now returned to where the sequence began, and so it is time to round off the healing by stepping back and making the energetic separation (see page 19).

Your patient will probably feel very relaxed and drowsy after this treatment and may like to be covered with a soft blanket for awhile to finish absorbing the healing. When ready, an offer of a glass of water or cup of tea is usually welcome. Try to end the session quietly, without too much conversation, before you and your patient move on to the tasks of normal living.

2. Two Healers, Patient Lying Down

It is supportive and can be stimulating to work with another healer to give a joint healing sequence to one patient. Giving a joint chelation is ideal for this.

The lead healer makes the decisions about when to move on to the next healing position. You and your fellow healer need to be intuitively aware of each other and to make eye contact after about two minutes at each position, so that you can indicate the next move and make it smoothly, together. The lead healer is responsible for initiating the eye contact while the fellow healer has to remain alert enough to sense when it's coming.

- When you've made your patient comfortable, decide with your cohealer which of you is going to be the lead healer for this sequence. Prepare individually, by grounding and running energy, and then stand facing each other and attune your energies by placing the palms of your hands together (right palm to left and vice versa).
- If you're the lead healer, you should stand at your patient's head with your fellow healer at your patient's feet. Having asked permission to lightly touch your patient's body, you, as lead healer, put both hands on your patient's head (as in the first exercise, page 135), while your fellow healer puts their right hand on the sole of your patient's right foot and left hand on the sole of your patient's left foot. As you and your fellow healer maintain the position at your patient's head and feet, you will probably become aware of energies flowing and balancing through your patient and of a strong contact with your fellow healer.
- Next you place your left hand at the base of your patient's neck on the right-hand side, and your fellow healer joins you at your patient's head and puts their left

hand beside your right hand, and right hand at the
right-hand base of your patient's neck.

- After about two minutes of healing flow, make eye
  contact with your fellow healer and, as synchronously as
  possible, move your right hand down to join your left
  hand while your fellow healer moves the left hand down
  to join the right. You then move your left hand to your
  patient's left shoulder and your fellow healer moves the
  right hand to your patient's right shoulder.
- After about two minutes, or when you sense a positive
  healing change, make eye contact with your fellow healer
  and move your right hand to join your left at the
  shoulder. When both sets of hands have been very
  briefly at the same point together, move your left hand
  down to your patient's left elbow, while your fellow
  healer mirrors your movement at the right side of your
  patient's body, with their hands complementing yours.
  At your side of the body, right hand follows left and at
  your fellow healer's side, left hand follows right. The
  hands should never cross over each other and the lead
  hand should not leave a chelation point until it has been
  joined, for a moment, by the following hand.
- Wait again, either for two minutes or until you sense
  change, make eye contact with your fellow healer and
  bring your right hand to join your left at the left elbow
  of your patient, while your fellow healer mirrors your
  movement, with opposite hands, on the other side of
  your patient. Move your left hand to your patient's left
  wrist while your fellow healer moves right hand to right
  wrist.

Now continue the sequence:

- After two minutes of healing flow, make eye contact with
  your fellow healer and bring your right hand to join
  your left at your patient's left wrist, then move your left

hand to your patient's left waist. Your fellow healer mirrors these movements, in unison, at the right side of your patient's body.

- After two minutes of healing flow and on eye contact with your fellow healer, your right hand joins your left at your patient's left waist, followed by moving your left hand down to your patient's lower hip while your fellow healer mirrors, in unison, on the right-hand side of your patient.

- After two minutes of healing flow and on eye contact with your fellow healer, your right hand joins your left at your patient's left lower hip and then your left hand moves down to your patient's left knee. On the other side of your patient's body, your fellow healer mirrors these movements in unison—left hand joining right at right lower hip and right hand moving to left knee.

- After two minutes of healing flow and on eye contact with your fellow healer, who mirrors your movements on their side of your patient's body, your right hand joins your left at your patient's left knee and then your left hand moves down to your patient's left ankle. (Fellow healer moves left hand to join right at right knee and right hand moves to right ankle.)

- After two minutes of healing flow and on eye contact with your fellow healer, who mirrors your movements in unison, your right hand joins your left at your patient's left ankle and your left hand moves down to the sole of your patient's left foot. (Fellow healer moves left hand to join right at patient's right ankle and right hand to the sole of your patient's right foot.)

- After two minutes of healing flow and on eye contact with your fellow healer, your right hand joins your left on the sole of your patient's foot and your fellow healer's left hand joins right on the sole of your patient's right foot.

- As lead healer, you now lift your left hand from your patient's right foot, but maintain contact with your right

hand, allowing your fellow healer to move their right
hand to join yours on the sole of your patient's left foot.
Once your fellow healer is in the position where their
right hand is on the sole of your patient's left foot with
their left hand still in contact with the sole of your
patient's right foot, you break your contact with
your patient's foot and walk quietly up the right-hand
side of your patient, back to the position at your patient's
head where you began the healing sequence. (You have
worked down the left side of your patient's body, but you
walk up the right side, back to the head.)

- Put both hands gently on the crown of your patient's
  head. Make a strong renewed attunement to your fellow
  healer with their hands on the soles of your patient's feet
  and then gently, in unison, release the contact and walk
  away. Make your energetic separation from your patient
  and also on this occasion make an energetic separation
  from your fellow healer and they from you.

Again, your patient will probably feel very relaxed and
maybe drowsy after this treatment. Remember to offer a
soft blanket and to allow time for them to finish absorbing
the healing. When ready, offer a glass of water or cup of
tea. Try to end the session quietly, without too much conversation, before you, your patient, and your fellow healer
move on.

If circumstances are such that your patient needs to sit on
a chair to receive a chelation, the movements and sequences
are the same and one healer can work alone or two healers
together. To achieve the position where your hands are
under the soles of your patient's feet, it's helpful if the
patient has their shoes off and has a foot cushion. (It has
been assumed that a prone patient would almost automatically have shoes removed.)

Working in the auric field, with your hands and healing chakras, energy points and subtle bodies, is the main substance of a healer's work, but there are other tools for healing that can be used alongside this basic knowledge to expand and enhance your healing sessions and bring special qualities and benefits to your healing interactions. The next chapter describes and explores some of these.

Chapter 7

Other Tools for Healing

Pauline's story—Considering using tools for healing—Color—
Crystals—Fragrances—Sounds—Helping others to help
themselves—Absent or distant healing—Exercises

PAULINE'S STORY

Like Robert (see page 114), Pauline was a natural healer
but she had very different difficulties. In some ways her
sensitivities were too open because she "tuned in" not only
when healing, but all the time. In everyday life, she found
it difficult to be near other people unless they were family
or very well known to her. She could not watch news
programs on television or read newspapers easily because
her extreme openness and psychic empathy made her feel
ill or depressed when learning of others' difficulties or
suffering. She knew she was a healer, but hesitated to practice as one because she became too moved by the thought
of her patient's pain or disease. Before she learned about
energetic separation, she picked up symptoms if she gave

anyone healing, and not just mildly and fleetingly but quite acutely, perhaps for several days.

When Pauline came to see me, she needed help and healing for herself as well as to resolve an energetic problem quite common among healers. I've often observed that unless healers express their ability to heal in some way they get intensifications and loop-backs of energy in their own subtle systems and find normal life trying, invasive, and tiring. Such people need help to control their sensitivities so that they know how to shut down without shutting off, while still being able to open up safely when it's appropriate. Their subtle body layers need strengthening and blending.

In a combination of healing and teaching, I introduced Pauline to the energetic separation exercise (see page 19) and encouraged her to use it for all kinds of purposes: to be less open to others when traveling on public transport or shopping; before watching television and during and after television programs; when reading the newspapers; as soon as she felt anything impinging on the sensitive feeling layer of her aura, and at any moment when she felt energy was beginning to drain from her. To do this, she had to learn to be aware that the energy drains and increased moments of sensitivity were happening, so that she could help herself before she became completely exhausted.

It's incumbent on all healers to develop a more acute awareness of what's happening to their own energies and to the energetic environment around them. Being sensitive should mean being aware and able to anticipate—and therefore take charge—of things. It should not mean being a victim of circumstance who's continually drained or over-affected by normal life. Sensitives need to be able to manage themselves well enough to participate fully in any and every aspect of life that they might wish to embrace.

Another exercise I taught Pauline to value and practice was the one designed to strengthen your energy field (see page 166), given toward the end of this chapter. It's similar to the exercise for enhancing your subtle body layers (see page 128), but has more emphasis on the use of personal, private, and public psychic space.

Pauline also needed to learn to give color to her own chakras so that the tone of their petals was enhanced and they could not flop open so easily and beyond her control. This was especially important for her at her heart chakra.

As she learned to be the one in control of her sensitivities, Pauline found she had more energy and began to enjoy a much fuller life. She also realized that she could practice healing without being drained psychically, emotionally, and physically. This was very empowering for her: if born healers practice healing, their own energies benefit and flow more naturally and healthily.

The new adjustments did not happen overnight. As Pauline began to give healing to others again, we looked in the first instance at methods of making the channeling less intensive for her. She found that visualizing and channeling color to patients was less taxing than merely opening as a channel for healing. She had a natural feeling for crystals and fragrances, and found that using these in a healing session left her more easily in control of her own sensitivities. (She also found crystals a great help when learning how to manage her own acute but delicate energy system.)

USING TOOLS FOR HEALING

There are specialist courses for healers who want to know a great deal about color, crystals, fragrances, and sound. But even without taking a formal course, these natural healing tools can be used effectively and safely by employing a little knowledge and a lot of feeling with extended awareness and intuition.

As a healer, it's a good idea to have a spectrum or palette of skills and alternatives. Not all will be appropriate all the time, and not all will attract you. For some healers, the tools mentioned here may feel like unnecessary appendages. For others, like Pauline, they can be a help in finding and defining a clearer and more comfortable relationship with healing energies themselves and with patients' needs and expectations. It's good to explore what's available, but also good to follow your own evaluation of what's, or is not, for you.

Using tools for the enhancement and variation of healing enables healers to use their skills, intuitions, and sensitivities in different ways. For example, when Pauline used color in various ways for healing her patients, she found that having this tool enabled her to become less enmeshed in the healing process and flow. Some of these tools can also be passed on to the patient to use for themselves between healing sessions.

COLOR

Because I believe the chakras to be basic in learning how to practice healing, color has already been an intrinsic part of the healing information in this book. It's extensively referred to in Chapter 5, where suggestions are included for visualizing color as you heal your patients.

In addition to learning to visualize and channel color, I would encourage healers to acquire simple color aids that can be used to enhance the healing environment and changed according to the needs of individual patients. Using color in your general home and life environment, and suggesting to patients that they use it in this way, is also important. Pauline found that using color helped her to help herself—it can be a fundamental aid to healers' own health and well-being.

As a nonprofessional healer, it's unlikely that you'll have a special room set aside for healing, but it's important to take as much care in preparing the environment as in preparing yourself for a healing session. That's not to say that a quick healing session on a kitchen stool or in the living room before you've cleared up the children's toys is any less effective in terms of transfer of energies, but having respect for your gifts and creating a whole and harmonious healing experience for your patients leads to a very different healer/patient relationship.

When you know that your healing skills are going to be called upon, try to arrange a time when you'll be free of other concerns. Prepare a space, even if it's only a corner of a room that's much used for other things, and employ color to help make that space harmonious.

As healing is mostly a heart-centered function, the colors of the heart chakra are good ones to consider. A pale green or rose cushion for your patient's feet, a green, rose, or amethyst-colored blanket or wrap to put around them during or after the healing sequence, a pink or green candle burning, a few heart-colored flowers in a suitable vase, or a green plant in the area will all help to create an atmosphere and enhance your attunement and your patient's receptivity.

If you're giving a series of healings to a patient with a particular need, you can vary some of these props accordingly. Add deeper rose colors for anyone who needs healing for a structural condition, such as rheumatism, arthritis, or back pain. Introduce some orange or amber for patients who need extra energy or who are anemic or rather depressed. Yellow and sunshine gold are helpful to digestive problems, while the heart colors help asthma, breathing difficulties, and oversensitivity. Blues are cooling where there is inflammation, and indigos and violets help eyes, head, and renewal of hope in life.

Remembering these touches will help your healing to be more specific to each individual and will add to your patients' sense of being seen, heard, and cared for. (There are fuller comments on color symbolism in Chapter 5.)

CRYSTALS

Full crystal healing is a discipline in itself, and there are courses and workshops available for those who want to learn in detail about crystals and their healing qualities. Each type of crystal (and, indeed, each individual crystal) has many different attributes. Studying these can open up whole new dimensions to your healing possibilities. Natural crystals, such as clear quartz, amethyst, rose quartz, and aventurine, to name but a few, are reminders to us of the spirit that resides in matter. Used as an aid to spiritual work and healing, crystals enhance and amplify.

At the simplest level, any healer can use crystals as a support to the healing process. An amethyst cluster in the space you use for healing will help to absorb and transform the difficulties that your patients bring in with them. The active healing energies contained in crystals are released when we declare our healing intention and use the crystal to help us focus on that intention or to help in directing the healing flow to a specific bodily area or chakra.

The chakra lists in Chapter 5 and the section here on page 151 give a range of crystals for each chakra, but broadly speaking, crystals are linked to chakras by their color. Red or dark crystals are for the root chakra and its associated functions, orangey ones for the sacral, yellow for the solar plexus, green for the heart, blue for the throat, indigo for the brow, and violet for the crown.

There are hundreds of different types of crystal, and deciding which to acquire can take some thought. It may help to remember that clear quartz points and rose quartz crystals are universal in their use and are particularly useful for healers who don't intend to acquire very specific or specialized knowledge of the use of crystals and gemstones in healing.

While some crystals are rare and fall into the pricey

gemstone category, many others are easily found at specialist or New Age shops, and often in market stalls. It's possible to acquire a small selection of simple but lovely crystals without breaking the bank. Once you've decided which varieties of crystal you'd like to acquire and found a source or supplier, rely on your intuition to select which of a particular variety is the right one for you and your healing practice.

Spend some time getting to know your crystal. Look at it carefully, handle it, and admire it. When you're ready to prepare your crystal for serious work, rinse it under running water several times, allowing it to dry naturally between rinses. Then, if possible, put the crystal on a piece of silk on a flat surface where it will catch as much light as is available, particularly sunlight. Leave it there for at least a day.

When the crystal has been cleansed and charged in this way, design a simple ceremony in which you dedicate it to its healing purpose. Light a candle and hold each stone in your cupped hands, asking that it may aid your healing work.

Without specific training with crystals, you'll only be using them as a support to your work. Because some people can be surprisingly anxious about the functions and powers of crystals, always ask your patient how they feel about your introducing crystals to the healing sequence or even into the healing space.

Using crystals can enhance the healing energies you're channeling and help in focusing them to specific areas. With your patient's permission, crystals can be placed or held on or near chakra points, disease points, or pain points. Use one crystal at a time, and unless you've had additional training or experience, don't place or hold them over the body, particularly the chakra points, for more than two consecutive minutes at a time.

Remember that crystals amplify, magnify, and focus other healing energies you're giving. As your hands may not be so active in the healing when you're using crystals, it's possible to overenergize (or overstimulate) a point or area. Trained crystal healers sometimes use many crystals and leave them lying on the body in special patterns or spreads, but if you're using crystals as a support to your normal healing practice, using one crystal energy at a time is easier to manage and monitor until your knowledge, experience, intuition, or special training with crystals is further developed.

If you have a few crystals on a shelf or in a basket, your patients can be encouraged to choose one to hold during a healing session or to put near their feet. This can be held or placed for the whole session since it's less involved in the direct healing flow.

Clear quartz points are single crystals of clear quartz with one pointed and faceted end and one flat or slightly rounded end. Such crystals can be very clear and beautiful, or have rainbows visible in them when you look into their centers. They can be used for any chakra and any purpose, but are particularly useful for combing the aura toward the end of a healing session. Aura combing is described in the exercise on page 37. It can be done with the tips of your fingers as you move your slightly splayed hands from the crown of your patient's head down to the feet, moving all around your patient as you do so. It can also be done with the pointed end of a clear quartz crystal, which has a particularly cleansing and soothing but energizing effect.

After a crystal has been used for healing, it should be washed under running water, dried, and left in a sunlit or lighted place until you're ready to use it again.

Crystals help to enhance intuition and creativity. If you decide to use them for healing, you should use your intuition to help you know when and which are appropriate to a particular patient or situation. Here, briefly, are the qualities of the crystals that were recommended for each chakra in Chapter 5.

Root Chakra

Agate strengthens our sense of purpose and brings a *joie de vivre*. It's helpful to those who fear poverty and deprivation, and it encourages abundance. It helps to strengthen parenting instincts and skills.

Bloodstone is purifying. It helps blood disorders.

Garnet and **alexandrite** are regenerative and help flesh and tissue to heal. They bring comfort to the bereaved and help generally in all times of loss or change.

Onyx gives strength and stamina. It's a good stone for those who feel overburdened by worldly responsibilities.

Rose quartz is a crystal for universal use. It's nurturing and brings a sense of unconditional love.

Ruby vitalizes, nourishes, and warms. It's the stone to use for healing when there's been a difficult birth, or bonding to the mother has been delayed for some reason.

Smoky quartz promotes calmness, centeredness, and groundedness. It helps to calm fear, panic, or shock.

Tiger's eye enhances creativity, protects in times of danger, helps when challenges have to be met, and aids fertility.

Sacral Chakra

Amber energizes, balances, and heals. It lifts depression, and aids dreams and creativity. It's useful for healing the female reproductive organs and for helping to regulate the menstrual cycle.

Aventurine helps to release blocked creativity and to activate the imagination.

Citrine heals wounded emotions and promotes emotional maturity. It helps where sexual problems and wounding have to be addressed.

Jasper is a stone of power and empowerment. It helps the oversensitive and those who have obsessional thought patterns.

Moonstone protects all who travel on water. It aids us in gaining contact with our feelings and in being able to see ourselves as others see us.

Topaz aids fertility and promotes inner peace.

Solar Plexus Chakra

Apatite aids concentration and intellectual thought, and the development of logical communication.

Calcite comes in many different colors. The orange, honey, and yellow varieties are most appropriate to the solar plexus and aid psychic development. They help to connect the higher will to the lower will.

Citrine is also mentioned at the sacral center. Bright yellow shades of citrine help in cultivating clarity, warmth, and a sense of self. It also helps the digestive system.

Iron pyrites aids all levels of assimilation and encourages the discovery of true potential.

Kunzite aids self-discipline, self-respect, and inner balance.

Malachite aids psychic and spiritual abilities, and the re-membrance of dreams. It's also healing for physical eyesight problems.

Rose quartz helps to keep the solar plexus flexible.

Topaz strengthens vision and purpose but also aids cheerfulness and humour.

Heart Chakra

Amber purifies the heart and aids the development of balance and love.

Azurite aids compassion and is helpful in healing allergies and asthma.

Chrysoberyl comes in many forms and colors, including the emerald. These stones are comparatively rare and rather expensive to acquire, but they attract kindness and generosity. They are revitalizing and therefore sometimes called the stone of perpetual youth.

Emerald helps to bring about that balance of heart and mind that leads to wisdom. It encourages the development of loyalty, trust, and love.

Green calcite heals the subtle bodies and particularly the feeling body. It heals wounds of the heart and helps to bring strength during periods of change or transition.

Jade (green or white) helps to regulate the heartbeat and to increase vitality, longevity, and life force. It also aids the development of serenity, wisdom, harmony, and perspective.

Tourmaline has a wide range of colors, including black. The rose and watermelon varieties are most suited to the heart chakra, where they aid tolerance, flexibility, compassion, and transformation. They promote harmony and being non-judgmentalism. They help the heart when it has to bear trauma, loss, or bereavement.

Throat Chakra

Aquamarine eases fears and phobias. It aids positive communication with large audiences and is therefore an excellent stone for writers, journalists, and people who work in the media.

Lapis lazuli aids expression of all kinds. It's helpful to the healing of deafness.

Sapphire is said to enable communication with other planets. It strengthens the throat chakra and nurtures the gift of prophecy, or channeling and mediumship.

Sodalite, which is often mistaken for lapis lazuli but lacks the gold spots that distinguish lapis, is excellent for healing all inflammatory throat conditions and the thyroid gland.

Turquoise aids the search for true purpose and enhances clarity in communication.

Brow Chakra

Amethyst enhances spiritual awareness and encourages vision. It's a protective stone and transforms negativity.

Azurite is an aid to rituals and blessing ceremonies because it enhances sacredness. It promotes visionary dreams and helps to harmonize the relationship between spirit and matter.

Blue fluorite is protective. It's a psychic shield, valuable in developing transcendent states of consciousness.

Calcite strengthens the higher mental body. It links the world of spirit with the world of intellect and ideas.

Pearl is for purification and also aids serenity and devotion.

Purple apatite stimulates all levels of perception and aids meditation.

Sapphire strengthens spiritual awareness and communication. It facilitates connection with guides and angels.

White fluorite strengthens the incarnate spirit and helps to prevent depression and disillusionment.

Crown Chakra

Celestite aids meditation and heals and fortifies the petals of the crown chakra. It awakens our desire to celebrate the spiritual aspects of life.

Diamonds are for perfection and clarity. They draw us toward our highest spiritual potential and encourage the higher will to illuminate the personality.

Snowy quartz heals resentment and loneliness. It strengthens the soul body but also encourages a feet-on-the-ground approach to life.

White jade awakens the inner divine spark and strengthens communication with the higher self.

White tourmaline encourages integrity and facilitates the deeper understanding of spiritual surrender and obedience. It promotes inner honesty and insight.

Alter Major Chakra

Carnelian encourages contact with nature spirits (see Glossary, page 189). It aids memory of previous lifetimes and the dreaming of positive dreams.

Fossils help us to connect with the wisdom stored in the collective unconscious (see Glossary, page 189). They promote a natural and relaxed approach to life, incarnation, and evolution.

Peacock stone (sometimes called bornite or chalcopyrites) aids the recall of skills known and practiced in another life-time. This particularly applies to remembering or reviving ancient healing skills.

Snowflake obsidian is linked to the cycles of life, death, and rebirth, and gives stamina for all times of change.

Tiger's eye enables greater contact with the earth and its rhythms and seasons. It will help herbs to grow in your herb garden, if shallowly "planted" alongside them.

FRAGRANCES

You'd rarely use fragrances directly to enhance your healing sequence at a first session with a patient, but in a general sense it can be helpful to have lavender fragrance in your healing space. This is calming, cleansing, and aids energetic separation (see page 19). As with all fragrances, you should aim for it to be subtly rather than powerfully present. A drop of lavender essential oil in a small bowl of water, a delicately fragranced lavender candle, or a fine spray of lavender water on the palms of your hands before you begin healing are all ways to bring fragrance into the space.

Cautions About Using Fragrances

True aromatherapy is a specialized form of healing and you should therefore use fragrance quite tentatively. Without specialist knowledge, refrain from using essential oils with women who are pregnant. If you intend to use fragrance in a session, you'll need to ask any woman patient of child-bearing age whether there's any possibility that she could be pregnant. (Lavender oil as part of the general ambience is excepted here.) You'll also need to check with your patient that they're not particularly susceptible or allergic to any aromas. It's a good idea to try out particular fragrances for yourself before using them with clients, so that you can judge how intense they may become.

Using Essential Oils

These considerations aside, once you get to know the nature of a patient's specific needs, the judicious use of a little fragrance, in the form of an essential oil, can be very beneficial to support the healing sequence. Essential oils are pure plant and flower extracts and are very concentrated. One of the best ways to use them in the healing environment is to burn just a drop or so in an oil burner or diffuser.

It's important to use the type of diffuser that allows you to float the oil on water. The oil itself should not be burned or heated directly. Overheating an oil can change its character and may alter the fragrance and its benefits. When using oils on your own hands, mix a drop or so of essential oil with a carrier oil, such as sweet almond or jojoba.

Although joss or incense sticks are available in most essential oil aromas, I don't recommend using these in the healing room. They often give off smoke, and the fragrance can become quite heavy and pervasive, especially in a small space. They can be good for cleansing a healing space before or after a healing, but avoid burning them during an actual healing sequence.

Essential oils also have links to chakras. When considering whether the gentle use of fragrance might or might not be beneficial for a patient, remember that there are stimulating and quieting oils for each chakra. As you learn to read chakras you'll often pick up a sense of under- or overactivity.

An overactive chakra feels excited and tingly or tense when attention is focused into it. Such a chakra may also be open and vulnerable. It needs calming and quieting, and one of the calming oils or a mixture of those recommended can be used to help this process. An underactive chakra will feel cold and closed. It'll be difficult to sense a response from it. It needs stimulating and encouraging. One of the stimulating oils for that chakra, or a blend of them, can be used to achieve this.

As you familiarize yourself with the essential oils, I'd encourage you to rely on your intuition about what to use and when to use it, although you should always take the precautions mentioned above into consideration. Use the fragrances in the environment around your patients or on your own hands as you heal gently on the body or in the auric field. Leave it to specifically trained people to put the oil-borne essences directly on the skin or to massage with them.

SOUNDS

The relationship of sound to healing is being constantly researched. Sound healing has also become a discipline in its own right, and you can attend workshops and courses to learn about it. However, you don't have to be trained in sound healing to consider using it to support your own healing practice if you use it in a gentle way and always consult your patient before doing so.

I've often discussed with healers on healing courses the issue of whether or not to play music during healing sessions. My own view is that taste in music can be very personal, that it's not always easy to reproduce it with good quality, and that it's difficult to know at what volume it becomes intrusive. If it's either too soft or too loud, it can become an irritant rather than an asset. I wouldn't choose to play music during a healing session or to have it played when I'm the one being healed. This is a personal viewpoint, and as with so many things, healers must eventually choose for themselves what works best for them and their patients, and be prepared to learn from experience.

I often play music to prepare myself before giving a healing session, or to help in preparing the healing space. Music of the Baroque period is conducive to healing vibrations and the slow movements from Mozart concertos have a particularly healing vibration. Apart from the classics, there is a wide variety of tapes and discs that have been prepared by intuitive, healing, and musical people. Explore the field, and sense what's right for you, and use it accordingly for your own meditation, for cleansing or preparing your healing space, and perhaps as you're making your healing attunement or rounding off for a patient.

Using Musical Instruments

A healing sequence that you might add to your repertoire is given in the exercise on page 168. For this you need to collect a selection of musical instruments, which could include a drum, rattle, rainstick, triangle, bell or singing bowl. The sounds these instruments make are cleansing and harmonizing to the subtle bodies and the chakras. The drum restores natural rhythms, the rattle helps to clear unwanted thoughts, the rainstick clears toxins and is particularly useful for people undergoing chemotherapy or radiotherapy, the triangle and bell are also cleansing and balancing, and the singing bowl helps people attune to their true selves and their chakras so that these balance individually and in relationship to each other.

Practice with any instruments you acquire until you're familiar with them and can make sounds that are reasonably controlled. With a drum you should be able to sustain a gentle, rhythmic sound that shouldn't be drummed more slowly than the normal heartbeat. Fast, loud drumming is a shamanic (see Glossary, page 190) healing practice and is best avoided unless you have specifically studied that area.

Rattles

Rattles are shamanic instruments. With practice you can shake one gently and consistently around your patient's aura or over chakras to help free the patient from worries or obsessions.

Rainsticks

These simply need rotating from end to end for their cleansing sound to flow. Be careful when selecting your rainstick that the sound made as the materials inside it flow from end to end is reasonably sustained and does not begin or end too abruptly.

Triangles

Although you might feel that triangles belong mainly to the grade school percussion band, they have a very pure sound that disperses and rebalances energy in the subtle bodies and around the chakras. Practice until you can strike yours accurately enough to get its clearest sound as often as possible. You can then strike it over organs or chakras to clear blockages, or in the auric field for cleansing and clearing.

Healing bells

A healing bell should be light and bright in tone. It's usually quite small and light in itself. Choose one that's pure and pleasant in its tone and it will function in healing in a similar way to the triangle.

Singing bowls

Singing bowls are not cheap to acquire. Some are old and some modern. When choosing, be guided by your own response to the sound. Generally, the larger the bowl the deeper the tone. True singing bowls are made of brass and come from Tibet. You need a simple, lathe-turned wooden striker or baton to strike them. This can be used in two ways.

While holding the bowl on the palm of your hand, but without any fingers touching its sides, gently strike the bowl two or three times with the baton. Because of the construction of the bowl, the sound will sing on and on and on.

Having started the resonance with the striker, you can then run it gently around the top of the bowl, with the striker held vertically and in touch with the bowl. It takes exploration and practice to be able to sustain this movement at the right speed and pressure. If you go too fast or have an uneven pressure, the striker will squeak against the bowl and interfere with the true resonant note.

When you become really expert at the movement of the striker around the top of the bowl, you won't need to strike the bowl to start the resonance but can simply move the striker around the bowl until it starts to sing and keeps on singing. Singing bowls can be sounded over chakras, organs, and in the auric field for purposes of harmonizing, cleansing, and balancing.

When to Use Musical Instruments

The sound chelation (draining of negative energy) is the main way to use sound to support your healing practice. But you can start and/or end a healing session with the chime of a bell or triangle, or the sound of a singing bowl. You can do the same thing at any time during a healing sequence, to aid clearance (but warn your patient beforehand that this might happen!).

You can use any instrument you may have available in your healing space, for a few moments, as your intuition guides you. Practice with a friend or partner to help you first, and note your reactions to the instruments. Sound is a serious, supportive, healing intervention, but have fun with it too!

HELPING OTHERS TO HELP THEMSELVES

One of the best ways of supporting your healing practice is to be aware of the tools that you can pass on to your patients, so they can further their own healing between sessions with you.

It's important that patients do not assume that having found a healer they can or must hand everything over to you. This is particularly relevant when people have a long-term illness or condition. Though the attitude in allopathic medicine toward patient participation in the healing process is gradually changing, it has tended to give us the message that we're wrong to want to be involved in the decisions made about treating our illnesses. However, engagement with our own healing journey is important.

Knowing that there are tools that can help us toward a positive outcome of disease helps us remain in a place of choice and autonomy. Your patients need you, and will put a lot of faith and hope in your abilities. From very early on in the healing process, it's good to hand back some of the responsibility to patients by asking them to work on themselves and their healing between sessions, and by reassuring them that they can do so effectively.

It's said that good teachers not only impart information but teach us how to learn. It might also be said that good healers not only impart healing but teach us how to heal ourselves.

Exercises That Patients Can Use

A number of the exercises given in this book are not only suitable for you as a developing healer, but are also applicable for your patients to practice, too, in the interest of self-healing. One of the most healing things for Pauline (see page 143) was to learn about energetic separation. It's not uncommon for many of us today to feel that the rush and crush of ordinary life impinges upon us in a way that adds to our stress, especially if we are ill or worried.

Energetic separation (see page 19) helps us maintain our own space. It can also be used to help us separate from difficult experiences—not in the sense of denying them, but in the sense of keeping a separate strength and wholeness with which to deal with them. I have known chemotherapy patients who've used energetic separation successfully to be able to say: "I am not the chemotherapy. The chemotherapy is not *me*. It is a treatment that will enable me to get well again."

Energetic separation can also be used to help in dis-identifying with an illness (not denying it). In the English language we have too many statements that say: "I *am* ill." "I *am* lame." "I *am* deaf." "I *am* angry." Such statements subtly imply that we are no more than our illness or our emotions. Consciously substituting *have* for *am* and using the energetic separation exercise can work remarkably to put us in a greater position of choice when it comes to managing the condition we have. We don't "become" a condition, and we don't have to lose contact with our true selves. We can always maintain choice and jurisdiction.

The exercise relating to analyzing illness and the sick self (see page 84) is one that patients can be encouraged to explore. It will help them understand more about the underlying dynamics of their illness and realize that making life and attitudinal changes are important to total healing and health.

The exercise for enhancing your subtle body layers (see page 128) can also be taught to patients. If they practice it at least once between sessions, their auras will become much more receptive to healing energy. Also, some of the balancing of colors and chakras will be in hand, so that your healing sessions can become more specific, direct, and immediate rather than having the supportive and general level take a major proportion of the healing time and energy. (This will automatically happen if your patients have done some self-work between sessions and therefore come to you with a more resilient aura.)

Two of the exercises later in this chapter are helpful to patients. The exercise on strengthening your energy field (see page 166) is as useful for patients as it is for healers, while the meditation exercise (see page 169) is specifically designed as a self-healing meditation.

Frequency of Healing Sessions

Some of your patients may come for one healing session only, while others may come for a series. Obviously, you will vary the frequency of healing sessions according to the patient and your own intuition, but usually they should not be more than once a week unless someone is very ill or has a short-term acute condition, in which case even daily healing can be appropriate. The spaces between healing sessions are important to healing absorption. Too much dependence on you as a healer should be discouraged in favor of helping your patients take more responsibility for self-healing. When the healer is redundant, the patient, hopefully, is well.

Preparing Tapes for Self Healing

In the early stages, patients may press for greater frequency once they feel that you're able to help them. Having a tape with a self-healing meditation, given in your voice, will help them have an interim connection with you, and also assist them in working toward their own healing. Reading the meditation exercise (see page 169) onto tape can be a start, but as you gain confidence you can design your own healing meditations and personal tapes for patients to encourage this important self-involvement.

Quite short tapes can be made to help patients relax. Taped instructions about feeding colors into appropriate chakras can be useful to encourage self-work between sessions. You might tape yourself talking a particular patient through a meditation at the beginning of a healing session and then offer the tape to be taken home and used between visits. Or you could make a tape of the induction for the color meditation exercise (see page 103) and the exercise at the end of this chapter (the induction is the first two paragraphs of the exercises). You might then suggest that your patient breathes some spring green and pink color into the petals of the heart chakra before moving on to another chakra or body part that you feel would benefit from color or attention.

Suggesting Crystals, Fragrances, and Sounds

You can introduce your patients to crystals and suggest they get one or two appropriate ones to have in their environment to remind them of a color useful to their general healing process. A crystal at the bedside can help patients remember to ask for healing before sleeping. You can also suggest that crystals be held over chakras or pain and disease points for a few moments each day—but emphasize that a maximum of five minutes is enough when holding a crystal over a chakra point, although they can be left on pain areas for longer. In addition, you can show patients how to comb their own auric field with a clear quartz point.

If your patients respond well to fragrances that you've introduced into the healing room or used on your hands when healing, you can suggest that they get a suitable essential oil and a carrier oil. Advise them to mix a few drops of essential oil into the carrier oil and then use this mixture as an addition to bath oils, as a skin fragrance, or for gentle massage of painful parts.

Patients with whom you've used sound might be keen to have one of the simple instruments mentioned above in their own homes. Listening to the true, clear sounds made by these is healing in itself and can clear an atmosphere or a mood.

Using Absent Healing

Finally, you can offer to put your patients on your absent healing (see page 165) list, particularly if you incorporate a practice of spending ten or twenty minutes daily or two or three times a week using this healing focus. Having a set time for them to "tune in" is helpful. I simply light healing candles at 9 pm each day and spend a quiet time remembering all those who've asked for healing flow and thought.

ABSENT OR DISTANT HEALING

Returning to my belief that all natural healers need to be involved in healing to be healthy in themselves, absent or distant healing is helpful if you don't have time, space, or inclination to heal patients directly. Pauline, for example, found it a help to do distant healing for and with friends before she felt strong enough to give hands-on healing.

Absent or distant healing works very well. Some of your patients may not be able to come to you for healing as often as might be desirable. Others may be family members or friends living at a distance. Arrange to have a quiet time in which you think or intuitively direct healing energy toward them or "hold them in the light." A group of you may gather together at a regular time to send out absent healing to individuals, to world leaders or causes, to animal, mineral, and plant kingdoms, and to the substance of earth itself.

Light a candle and maybe have a favorite crystal beside you. Do the grounding and running energy practice. Make a healing invocation, including in this the angels of light and love and healing.

Say aloud, three times, the name of the person for whom you're requesting healing, without saying why they require the healing or dwelling on any symptoms you know them to have. Imagine that person surrounded with golden light. After about three to five minutes of focus and concentration, see your distant healing patient fit, well, and following their favorite pursuits.

You can extend and amplify this healing ceremony by lighting a small candle or night light for each person or concern to which healing is being sent. At the end, as you extinguish the light or lights, think of the light being sent out rather than putting a candle out. See streams of light flowing toward those to whom healing has been given and see them as whole and healthy.

It's best to get people's permission before sending them absent healing, but since this is general rather than specific healing—a holding in light rather than a defined intervention—you can also use it for those who are too ill to make a personal request or where others have requested healing for a loved one.

Exercise
Strengthening Your Energy Field

This exercise helps to develop and strengthen your energetic temple of being, which defines personal, private, and public space.

- Making sure that you'll be undisturbed, sit or lie in a comfortable but symmetrically balanced position. Wrap yourself in a blanket for comfort and warmth if you wish, remembering that in meditation your body may lose heat. Unless you're sitting cross-legged or in a lotus position, don't cross your legs at the ankles or knees. Don't fold or cross your arms. Have the palms of your hands open and curved, and facing upward. You can balance your hands, palms open and up, on your knees if you're sitting, and on the floor or couch beside you if you're lying.
- Be aware of the rhythm of your breathing—don't force your breath or try to calm it. Simply allow it to find its own natural rhythm. Gradually bring that rhythm into your heart center or chakra, and sense how each in-breath and out-breath feeds, relaxes, and opens your heart chakra.

- Enter your inner space and imagine yourself sitting at a central, beautiful, peaceful place within a larger temple. This is your inner sanctuary, and you can spend some time creating it and making it just as you want your inner sanctuary to be. Beyond the inner sanctuary there are many courtyards, each of which is associated with a different color. Your inner sanctuary will be white, gold, silver, or violet in essence, but you can also add any other favorite colors.

- Your sanctuary is sacrosanct, and none may enter here unless you invite them specifically. There'll probably be very few to whom you would extend that invitation. Your guardian angel (see Glossary, page 188) helps you guard this sanctuary and to maintain its inviolability.

- Move out of your sanctuary to explore the courtyards. Those near your sanctuary are open only to people or influences you know and trust, and those further away are open to the potential for new acquaintances and new experiences. By filtering these through the courtyards and meeting them always outside your actual sanctuary, you protect yourself from invasion, give yourself time for assessment of others, and also make sure that you're being seen as you want to be seen. There may be an association with elements in the courtyards or with music, poetry, art, and fragrance.

- Enjoy creating and exploring your inner sanctuary. Return to it whenever you feel vulnerable. Know that there's always a central space that's yours and yours alone, and that you can keep other concerns and meeting places in the courtyards most appropriate to them.

- Return to the breath in your heart chakra and to your awareness of your body. Put a cloak of light with a hood right around you and return, without rushing, to your everyday world and tasks.

Exercise
Drawing Out Negative Energy Using Sound

For this healing sequence, choose an instrument from those mentioned above with which you're familiar and which you've practiced using beforehand.

To draw out negative energy (see page 134), move around the patient paying attention to energy points at the head, the feet, and at the main joints of the body. For sound chelation the principle is the same, but you make sounds with your chosen instrument over the energy points and also around the body as you move between the energy points.

- Have your patient either lying down or sitting up. Do your grounding and running energy preparation (see page 16).
- Standing at the patient's feet, rattle gently at the crown of your patient's head (if you're using a rattle, for example), then pause before rattling down the left side of the head to the base of the neck.
- Rattle at the base of the neck, pause, and then rattle out to the left shoulder, rattle over the left shoulder, pause, and then rattle down to the left elbow.
- Rattle over the left elbow, pause, and rattle down to the left wrist. Rattle over the left wrist, pause, and rattle in to the left waist.
- Rattle over the waist, pause, and rattle down to the point where the left leg joins the body. Rattle over this point, pause, and rattle down to the left knee.
- Rattle over the left knee, pause, and rattle down to the left ankle. Rattle over the left ankle, pause, and rattle down to the sole of the left foot. Rattle over the sole of the left foot, pause, and rattle over to the sole of the right foot.

- Rattle over the sole of the right foot, pause, and rattle to the right ankle. Rattle over the right ankle, pause, and rattle up to the left knee. Rattle over the left knee, pause, and rattle up to the point where the right leg joins the body.
- Rattle over this point, pause, and rattle up to the right waist. Rattle over the right waist, pause, and rattle out to the right wrist. Rattle over the right wrist, pause, and rattle up to the right elbow.
- Rattle over the right elbow, pause, and rattle up to the right shoulder. Rattle over the right shoulder, pause, and rattle up to the right-side base of the neck.
- Rattle over the right-side base of the neck, pause, and rattle up to the crown of the head. Rattle over the crown of the head, pause, and rattle down the center of the body to the feet. Rattle over the feet, pause, and rattle up the center of the body back to the crown of the head.
- Rattle once more over the crown of the head, put your instrument down, and make your energetic separation (see page 19).

Exercise
Using Meditation to Heal Yourself

This is a good exercise to promote your own health as a healer (see Chapter 8). It's also a good one to teach your patients and can be used as an absent healing meditation, where you hold others in the rainbow light.

- Make sure that you're not going to be disturbed. If possible, light a candle and dedicate it to your healing. Sit or lie in a comfortable, symmetrical position and become aware of the rhythm of your breathing. Within the breath rhythm become aware of your heart chakra.

Feel the petals of your heart chakra opening, allowing the heart energy to flow.

- Travel on the heart breath into your inner space and imagine yourself walking along a wooded pathway. The ground is soft under your feet and the fragrance of leaf mold is around you. Sun is dappling through the trees and you can hear the sound of moving water.

- Soon, through the trees, you see a busily babbling stream and you walk toward it. You decide to follow the stream, walking in the direction from which it's flowing. As you come out of the wood, the ground is drier and quite stony. You're going gently uphill. Now there are some bigger rocks around you, and you become aware of a waterfall somewhere near. You come upon the waterfall rather suddenly. It's splashing down from some higher rocks into a natural pool, from which the stream runs. The sun is shining and a misty spray rises from the water. In the sunlight, the spray is full of rainbows.

- You find a smooth rock, which has been warmed by the sun. As you sit on it, you realize that you're being bathed in rainbow healing light. Sit for a while and let the light flow over and into you. Feel it going to any place where there's pain or unease. Feel the vitality that it brings. When you feel ready, you'll get up and make your way back alongside the stream to the wooded path where this journey began.

- Before you leave the place of the waterfall, wash your hands and perhaps drink from the clear water in the pool. In the depth of the pool, there may be a gift for you—a symbol to help you on your healing path.

- After your return to the wooded path, become aware of the rhythm of your breathing and of your heart center. Enter the outer world once more. Blow out your candle. Let the flower of your heart center close in a little and visualize a cross of light in a circle of light as a blessing over it.

This chapter has introduced ideas and practices that may be more appropriate for the more experienced healer running a healing practice for patients other than family and friends, but it's always a good idea to aim for a professional standard, even in informal surroundings and with people you know well. If you want to expand beyond working with family and friends, there are practical and professional considerations you'll have to address. The next chapter on the health of the healer looks at some of these, and at the important transition from nonprofessional healer to fully practicing professional healer.

Chapter 8

Becoming a Professional Healer

Keeping it simple—Practical considerations—Who heals the healer?—Will I need some allied skills?—Referral to other agencies—Keeping well in body, mind, emotions, and spirit— Using meditation

KEEPING IT SIMPLE

Having started with a simple approach to healing, it may seem that more structure and more knowledge bring more complexity. Most healers I've known and worked with become fascinated by the whole complex and absorbing subject of healing. They keep learning more and more, both from their own experience and from teachers of healing. Yet, having tried many healing sequences or different types of intervention, they almost invariably return to something quite simple and direct.

As one healer said to me: "There is a place for doing things with crystals and sounds and different energy points, but mostly I just want to be clear and simple and channel the energy that I know I can bring through me." I agree entirely, but also maintain that the simplicity that comes at the end of the journey is different from the simplicity that makes the journey necessary. The simplicity of a certain naïveté can be beautiful and direct, but the simplicity that is also informed is like a clear well-spring arising, full of nutrients, from the depths.

The journey to greater knowledge may also awaken in you the desire to be more than a healer for family and friends, and to look for further training, with the aim of having a professional practice where people pay for your services. If this is the journey you want to take, there has perhaps not been a better time to take it. There are many outlets and opportunities, but also professional and practical considerations.

PRACTICAL CONSIDERATIONS

Once you move into the professional field, having a healing corner at home, or knowing you can clear a suitable space when required, is not enough. You need somewhere more permanent, or you may want to hire a room for a few sessions in a natural health center.

When you're considering wider and more professional practice, the question of responsibility in the wider sense arises. This is more than mere loyalty and wanting to do the best for your patients. You'll need insurance. To get this you must belong to a healing organization or have gained a recognized healing qualification.

You cannot really be paid until you have some kind of professional standing, but in my experience, healers have great difficulty with the subject of payment and so I'd like to set out some considerations here. Even with family and friends, it's a good idea to have some kind of barter or exchange. This is a boundary issue. Difficulties always arise if one person is the constant giver and the other the receiver.

If there's a meaningful exchange, the patient feels freer to ask for a repeat treatment and the healer is less likely to feel a draw from or incursion into their time and space.

Of course, healing is an energy, not a medicine. It's freely available within the structure of the universe, not manufactured and packaged. Of itself, it cannot be priced. Yet if you're to heal as more than a hobby, to a point where perhaps you need to leave your job, reduce your working hours, or spend considerable time away from your family commitments, then the time you give to the work has to be valued, as is any professional's time. Doing courses can be expensive. It's reasonable to expect that these could be funded from your healing practice once it gets more serious.

Money, in our times, is a convenient form of exchange. If you receive a service, then you expect to pay for it in some way. So, once you feel you're professional, look at what your needs are and set an appropriate fee for healing by the hour or half-hour. If you don't absolutely have to earn from the healing, it still benefits those who receive to be able to give or return something. Some healers put out a donation bowl or a charity box.

WHO HEALS THE HEALER?

One of the benefits of courses and training is that healers meet each other, form friendships, and sometimes heal each other or give each other support. If you're a lone healer, try to find a group that you can sometimes meet or work with, where skill and support are shared.

Counselors and therapists are always expected by their professional organizations to be in supervision. This does not mean that they're perpetual students or probationers but that, because of the complexity of the issues and the relationship that can arise between counselor/therapist and client, there needs to be someone who can advise, support, and help in keeping a perspective, with confidentiality honored and protected.

I'd like to see more healers using this sort of consultation. Dealing with people who are ill, perhaps with serious diseases, perhaps facing death, can be a heavy weight to carry. Supervision gives healers a point of reference and support, and helps them to debrief and maintain a necessary warm detachment from some of the problems patients bring.

WILL I NEED SOME ALLIED SKILLS?

Many patients want to tell their experiences in full, and having them heard can be an important part of the healing process. Working with the symbolism of disease (Chapter 4) can be very helpful, as can designing meditative exercises and affirmations as part of a self-help program. Ideally then, healers should consider developing some counseling or listening skills.

You don't have to be a full-fledged counselor, but knowing the most helpful ways of listening to and drawing a patient out can be a bonus. Acquiring some facility in this area will also help you in knowing when it might be a good idea to suggest to a patient that they have some sessions with a therapist or counselor. Courses in these skills are usually readily available at local colleges of education.

Some healers train in one of the complementary skills, such as reflexology, aromatherapy, or massage, and let their healing skills flow through the discipline of the treatment. For some patients such therapies are more easily acceptable and less challenging than the thought of energy or spiritual healing.

REFERRAL TO OTHER AGENCIES

Referral to other agencies is an issue that healers should keep in mind. Once you're working with people who are not well known to you, it's wise to upgrade your knowledge of basic first aid and of symptoms that need medical attention (see Appendix, page 185). Practicality and healing must go side by side, if healers are to be respected. If there has been an accident, it's good to be channeling healing while basic first aid is done, but not good to be doing nothing but channeling healing when urgent mouth-to-mouth resuscitation is required.

Healers often have patients who are seeking energy or spiritual healing as a last resort, having tried everything else and there being no further medical treatment possible. More and more, though, people come to healers before this sad stage is reached. They seek the support of healing while receiving other, more conventional treatments. I've often worked with cancer patients who appreciate healing and counseling as aids to minimizing the unpleasant side effects of radiotherapy or chemotherapy.

Patients should always be supported in the choices they make about management of their illnesses. They should be encouraged to see their doctors, not discouraged. Healing is not an alternative therapy, but a complementary one. Many doctors are open to it and welcome the information that their patients are also seeing a healer for support. Some medical practices have healers available at the office or clinic for those patients who want this.

Always try to persuade your patients to tell their doctors that they're receiving healing. As you become more highly trained and professional, you should consider always asking your patients' permission for you to inform other practitioners that their patients are working with you.

KEEPING WELL IN BODY, MIND, EMOTIONS, AND SPIRIT

Most healers, especially when they're healing on a regular basis, feel well and are full of energy in themselves. Having the opportunity to channel healing is as vital to a healer as is the opportunity to run for a dedicated runner (as we have seen in Pauline's story, see page 143). Pauline's oversensitivity was partly due to the nature of her giftedness, but once she understood the principle of energetic separation, she realized that she could more easily manage her own energies as long as she could practice her healing.

This situation of potential imbalance of energies in a healer who has no opportunity to heal, who has resistance to being a healer, or who has not recognized the gift as such, is not a question of healing sapping the healer's own vitality. One of the questions most frequently asked by patients after a healing is, "Does it drain you?" The answer to this should be an emphatic "No." Healing energy is a channeled energy, with the healer naturally having the special sensitivities that allow that to happen or having developed them through training.

As a healer you're constrained to heal because it's what you are for, or about. You don't have to be a hands-on healer to satisfy that urge to heal. Many healers at work in our society would not call themselves healers in the way the word *healer* has been used in this book.

From Congress to courts of law, in schools and hospitals, in therapy rooms, in the business of everyday life, on buses and trains, in offices, shops, and bars, in homes and families everywhere, healers abound. Their leadership, justice, caring, ability to listen, sense of humor, quiet presence or creation of harmony has that extra ingredient of healing— you feel better for having seen, traveled with, or visited them. Such are the "hidden" healers in society who consciously or unconsciously have found a satisfying way to express what they have. They are rarely subject to energetic discomfort.

Realizing that you're a healer uncomfortable with your own sensitivities, but with no opportunity to develop your gift, may mean that you have to seek other ways of channeling healing than the hands-on variety. There are ways of managing and sublimating until you can make the life changes that may be necessary to honor your gift. Whatever you're involved in and cannot change, you can do it in a more healing way or from a more healing perspective.

I was a reluctant school teacher. When I eventually realized that I wanted to heal, not teach, I felt even more dissatisfied. Being a single parent with a young child meant that there were practical reasons why I couldn't easily change my life at that point. It was only when I realized that I could still see myself as a healer, although I needed to go on teaching for a while longer, that I adjusted more smoothly to my teaching career than I ever had before.

Others around me in my professional life probably noticed little, if any, change—I continued to teach as before. But for me, things changed a lot. I sought opportunities to make the teaching environment a healing one and to bring implicit healing into my relationships with staff, children, and parents. I created a different ambience in the classroom with color and the arts. I tried to let the healer flow through the teacher, rather than seeing the teacher as repressing the healer.

A friend of mine also longed to work with healing and was particularly interested in the healing use of color. Again, there were practical considerations preventing her from leaving her rather boring office job. Although stuck in an office, once she identified herself as a healer she found ways to bring in color, harmony, plants, and flowers. Suddenly her coworkers began to remark that they enjoyed coming to the office, because its atmosphere was so cared for.

In keeping well as a healer, the first consideration, then, is to respect and name yourself "healer." This opens the gateway to find expression for your true self, and to gain satisfaction from so doing.

A second consideration is to own the sensitivity you have so that you better learn how to manage it. Many sensitives say, "I don't want to become, or to seem, precious." In fact, the more you take care of and make provision for your sensitivities, the more normally you can function in everyday life. If you do nothing to manage your susceptibilities, then you'll become easily exhausted, bothered by crowds, and over-stressed by daily living. The energy exchange can be important to the healing flow and needs serious consideration. If you heal too often in your spare time, you'll become unable to sustain what you've set out to do. One thing healers must learn to avoid, in every sense, is getting stressed—burning the candle at both ends.

The management is very simple:

1. **Remember to ground and run energy at least once a day,** whether you're about to be involved in giving hands on healing or not (see page 16).
2. **Remember and understand the principles of energetic separation** and use them frequently (see page 19).
3. **Allow time for yourself.** As others become aware that you're a healer, they may expect you to "turn it on" at a moment's notice. Except in real need, try never to do this. If you've gone out for an evening or if friends have come to you, it's unwise to suddenly mix a healing session with a social occasion unless it's been previously arranged.

Such happenings make boundaries unclear and a healer's sensitive constitution needs clear boundaries. "Yes, I'll willingly give you some healing tomorrow at 10 A.M." is a more appropriate response to the spur of the moment request than to put your prospective patient on a stool in the midst of a crowded kitchen and give healing immediately. If you're socializing, socialize. If you're healing, set proper boundaries and keep it as a separate activity.

4. **Never imagine that putting strong shields of light around you and staying vulnerable inside them is the way forward.** You need strong and supple subtle bodies, and strong chakras that close and open their petals with ease, neither staying too tightly closed, nor being overblown and too full in their opening.

This means that you need to practice not only the central column breathing (see page 16) but also to feed your individual chakras with their "home" colors (red for the root, orange for the sacral, yellow for the solar plexus, green for the heart, blue for the throat, indigo for the brow, violet for the crown, and brown for the alter major). Practice the subtle body enhancing exercise (see page 128) and cleanse your etheric field (see page 130).

5. **Keep a balance in your life.** Have ordinary, mundane fun, enjoy creature comforts and celebrate your normality as well as your special gifts.

6. **Resolve to learn more about meditation** and bring some meditational practices into your life (see page 169).

7. **Take care of your own health and well-being** in every possible way. It is a myth that healers have to be complete models of good health, perfectly free from difficulties of their own and free from disease or tendency to disease. Generally, you need to feel vital and alert enough to be able to channel healing energy toward someone else. If you have an infectious cold, cough, or other transitory illness, it's best not to be in the close contact with patients that healing requires. When you're ill, get healing from your fellow healers and where necessary use medical treatment. The grounding and energetic separation exercises (see pages 16 and 19) will help to keep you in good health, as will the self-healing meditation (see page 169).

USING MEDITATION

Most healers have a natural aptitude for meditation and inner journeying, and experience slightly altered states of consciousness when giving healing. Even if you don't consider yourself to be a natural, the art of inner exploration can be developed with time and patience.

Once commonly practiced mainly in Eastern religions, meditation has become increasingly recognized in the Western world for its health-giving, stress-relieving, and creativity-enhancing benefits, as well as for spiritual attunement and to assist in the search for mystical experience. Yet confusion still arises as to what exactly meditation is. Essentially, it's an altered state of consciousness in which a range of subtle physiological and mental changes help to bring about a feeling of serenity. Some industrial companies provide opportunities for personnel to learn meditation so that the burdens of decision-making may be eased and new, creative ideas come from a place of inner peace.

The practices by which the meditative state is achieved are often confused with the state itself. Alternate nostril breathing, breath counting, breath watching, visualizing a rose, or chanting a mantra while watching a candle flame are all means to an end.

In the meditative or ruminative state we become receptive, our perceptions are subject to delicate change, and the less conscious reaches of our beings are more easily accessible. Thoughts, feelings, memories, images, and symbols, which may have been partially or wholly hidden, gently come to the surface to be recognized, owned, and examined, while the meditative state enables a centeredness and nonattachment that helps us to know truths about ourselves while maintaining an inner equilibrium.

The healer who acquires the discipline to practice meditation regularly acquires the ability to center and focus. When healing, a knowledge of meditation enables outer concerns to be left aside quickly so that the perceptions of healing can be experienced clearly and attended to effectively.

If you have some regular practices as a healer, such as grounding or meditation, you'll support your own healer identity and strengthen your subtle energy field, but discipline is an interesting subject in itself. I believe it should be gently acquired rather than rigorously enforced. Too much pressure renders the psyche resistant or defensive.

Establish a rhythm for your own spiritual practice that's comfortable and manageable alongside the other commitments in your life. Try not to make demands on yourself that are phrased along the lines of: "Every morning at 7 o'clock, I will always meditate and practice my grounding exercises." The day or life phase will inevitably come when you fail to meet your appointment with yourself and a "failure seed" may be sown.

If you take the attitude that, whenever possible, you'll meditate each day at a time that's regular but fits in easily with the rest of your life, then each time you keep an appointment with yourself and your support for your healer identity, you'll be sowing the seeds of success. Your practice will then grow regular for positive reasons and will bring you joy rather than coming from a rigorously imposed or artificial self-requirement.

Guided journeys and inner explorations require, but also facilitate, a slightly altered state of consciousness in which the focus of attention is inwardly directed. Progressively, they help us become more familiar with what is inside—or what is often termed the inner landscape.

You might like to make a tape recording of some of the longer meditative exercises or explorations given in this book. Leave appropriate pauses, so that you can play the tape to yourself as you meditate or journey without having to remember long sequences. If you tape the meditation, you can also time it and so know exactly how long you need to set aside. Then you don't need to become anxious about losing track of time.

At the beginning of each meditation, you're advised to make sure you'll be undisturbed. It's common for the body to lose heat in meditation, so wrap yourself in a blanket for warmth and comfort, or have one at hand in case you need it.

A standard cross-legged or lotus position is excellent for meditation. Your body forms a natural pyramid shape and the subtle energies flow well while being contained. If you are not comfortable in either of these positions and prefer to sit more normally on a cushion, on the floor, on a straight chair or armchair, or to lie down on the floor or a bed, it's important not to cross your legs at the knees or ankles. Have your body symmetrically arranged in a way that's relaxed and comfortable.

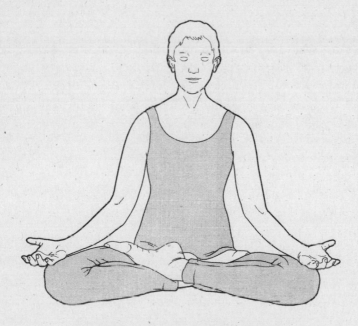

The lotus position used in meditation.

Keeping the legs uncrossed when sitting or lying other than in a true cross-legged or lotus position allows energy to flow freely without blockage or crossed polarities. For the same reasons, you shouldn't cross or fold your arms. Have the palms of your hands open and your fingers together but curved and facing upward. Balance your hands, palms open and up, on your knees if you're sitting, and on the floor beside you if you're lying down. This hand position helps you to be energetically balanced but receptive.

In the induction to each inner journey in this book, you're guided to open up your heart center or chakra. The heart energy is a particularly safe and wise energy on which to travel. Activating it ensures that your experiences will be vivid but gentle. If you visualize folding in the petals of your heart chakra as a protection at the end of a meditative visualization (see Meditations Using Color, page 103), that will help to make the transition between inner and outer worlds. The folding is soft, leaving the petals flexible and the chakra open enough to normal life without being either tightly shut down or wide open and vulnerable.

Meditation and inner visual practice is useful to healers. From your own practice of meditation and visualization, you'll gradually gain enough confidence to give your patients short inner exercises to aid self-healing and to sustain them between healing sessions (see Chapter 7).

May you and your healing flourish and this book have proved useful in helping you to be the healer you'd like to be.

Appendix

Symptoms Needing
Medical Referral

Cardiovascular
Chest pain during exercise
Blackouts
Ankle swelling and shortness of breath

Respiratory
Persistent chest pain
Shortness of breath
Coughing up blood
Weight loss
Prolonged wheezing attacks

Gastrointestinal
Vomiting blood
Passing blood from the rectum
Passing a sticky, black bowel movement
Persistent diarrhœa, especially with blood and slime
Abdominal pain, especially with vomiting and nausea
Change of bowel habit
Weight loss
Jaundice

Genito-urinary
Passing blood in the urine
Burning pain on passing urine
Severe loin pain
Men
Discharge from the penis
Difficult flow or inability to pass urine
Women
Abdominal pain during intercourse
Vaginal bleeding after intercourse, between periods, and after menopause
Breast lump
Urinary incontinence, especially when coughing or laughing
Acute abdominal pain with missed menstrual period

Hormonal
Weight loss, palpitations, tremor, protruding eyes
Weight gain, lethargy, coarsening hair and skin
Thirst, weight loss or gain
Infertility

Neurological
Double vision
Headache with nausea and vomiting
Weakness of limb function
Blackouts

Rheumatology
Severe pain over the temples with pains in the neck and shoulders (in rheumatology patients, these symptoms may lead to blindness)

Skin
Pigmented moles increasing in size
Pigmented moles with irregular outline
Pigmented moles with variable pigment density

Pigmented moles with itch or bleeding
Lesions on the face, especially in eye, nose, and cheek area

Eyes
Painful red eyes
Sudden loss of vision

Ears, nose, and throat
Fleshy swelling within the nostril
Prolonged pain in any of these areas
Hearing loss

Orthopedic
Acute bone pain at a specific site
Hip pain or limp in children
Curvature of the spine

Glossary

Akasha/ether. This is usually considered to be a fifth element. There's a progression from the tangible earth, water, fire, and air to the intangible akasha, or ether. It is like a collective energy body for humanity, holding the imprint of everything each individual, group, family, or race has ever known, done, or is in the process of knowing and doing. It is also thought to have a relationship to the origins of sound and color. Akasha is approximately the same as that which Jung described as the collective unconscious. Ether is not related to the chemical element but to the term "the ethers," which is sometimes used to describe other energetic planes.

Angels. Angels are direct reflections of Divine Consciousness. They're intermediaries and guardians helping the divine plan to manifest on earth.

The elemental/devic/angelic hierarchy or lifestream may be seen as moving from the Divine Consciousness toward earth, while the human stream of consciousness, which includes discarnate guides, may be seen to be moving toward reunification with the Divine. The elemental/devic/angelic hierarchy is therefore separate from humanity. Discarnates are not angels, and angels will not take on human form or consciousness.

Altered state (of consciousness). Electrical cycles in the brain can be measured. When we're dealing with everyday functioning and the material world, there is a normal range of cycles, known as the beta rhythms. When we sleep, we're mainly in theta rhythm. When, in waking consciousness, we're being particularly creative, alpha rhythms may be present. Through meditation or hypnosis we may enter altered states, in which beta rhythms fade, while alpha, delta, and theta rhythms become more constant. In such states our physical bodies relax, and we're more open to healing and may have an expanded awareness in which the barriers of time and space are lessened.

Drugs may induce altered states, but the cumulative side effects and other factors that often accompany drug-taking make them undesirable and usually counterproductive in any serious spiritual exploration.

Archetypes. By dictionary definition, these are "primordial images inherited by all." Each human society is affected by forces, such as peace, war, beauty, justice, wisdom, healing, death, birth, love, power. (These are sometimes called the archetypes of higher qualities.) The essence of these defies definition and we need images, myths, symbols, and personifications to help us understand their depth and breadth. Tarot cards, which have ancient origins, have twenty-two personified or symbolized archetypes in the major arcana. These cover all aspects of human experience. (*See also* Tarot.)

Bach Flower Remedies. Edward Bach, a doctor in the last century, discovered that sun-potentized essences of flowers could be produced and would work subtly to heal individuals and their emotional and physical illnesses or conditions. He produced thirty-eight flower remedies. Still popular today, they're available from most health-food stores, together with leaflets explaining their properties and uses.

Collective unconscious. This term comes from the work of C.G. Jung, the psychologist. It refers to the collective bank of human experience. Everything presently happening in our world affects us, although we are consciously aware only of our own little patch. Moreover, everything that has ever been experienced or accomplished by humanity, historically, is also stored. Myths and symbols can help us tap into the creative collective unconscious. Nightmares, anxieties, and irrational fears may be activated by collective rather than personal factors.

Higher self. Our higher self is, in essence, the part of our consciousness or soul that does not incarnate. The higher self has an overview of all our lifetimes and decides our task and purpose in each incarnation.

Nature spirits. These are tiny beings generally associated with plants, trees, the natural environment, and the elements. They are sometimes called elementals. They appear to those who have clairvoyant vision as points of light or color, or in traditional fairy form as nereids, sylphs, gnomes, elves, undines, goblins, and flower fairies.

Since the four elements interact in our physical bodies and largely determine our health patterns, nature spirits are within and around us. The giving and receiving of energetic healing activates and encourages them to help us to health and harmony.

Shamanic/shamanism. This refers to a tradition and healing form that originated in Iceland and parts of Russia, and also came to be practiced by the North and South Native Americans. Shamans undergo rigorous training that enables them to become seers and healers, and in full consciousness to cross the boundaries between the planes. Neoshamanism is a reawakening of the shamanic tradition.

Tarot. The Tarot is an ancient form of cards that can be read for the purposes of divination. The seventy-two cards comprise the major and minor arcana. The major arcana consists of twenty-two archetypes covering all aspects of human experience. The minor arcana has four suits, differently named in different versions of the cards, but mostly representative of mind, body, emotions, and spirit—or earth, air, fire, and water. The twenty-two archetypes of the major arcana are: the Fool, the Magician, the High Priestess, the Empress, the Emperor, the Hierophant, the Lovers, the Chariot, Strength, the Hermit, the Wheel of Fortune, Justice, the Hanged Man, Death, Temperance, the Devil, the Tower, the Star, the Moon, the Sun, Judgment, and the World.

Transpersonal therapy and counseling. This term addresses the spiritual and behavioral needs and aspirations of human beings. It concentrates on the importance of finding a meaning in life and of being creative and fulfilled in living, relating, and making choices.

Index

About the Author

Ruth White, U.K.C.P., is a transpersonal psychotherapist and spiritual teacher who conducts workshops throughout Britain and Europe. She is the author of several books and a founding member of Training for Supervisors at the Centre for Transpersonal Psychology in London.